Natural Solutions
For Sexual Enhancement

*Increase the energy in your sex life
with alternatives to drug therapy*

by

Dr. Howard Peiper
and
Nina Anderson

**Foreword by Harvey Diamond,
author of *Fit For Life*.**

Cover illustration by Albert Benoist

Published by
SAFE GOODS
East Canaan, CT

Natural Solutions For Sexual Enhancement
by
Dr. Howard Peiper and Nina Anderson

ISBN 1-884820-42-5
Library of Congress Catalog Card Number 98-61668
Printed in the United States of America

Natural Solutions for Sexual Enhancement is not intended as medical advice. It is written solely for informational and educational purposes. Please consult a health professional should the need for one be indicated.

Published by SAFE GOODS
283 East Canaan Rd.
East Canaan, CT 06024
(860)-824-5301

Table of Contents

DEDICATION

♥This book is dedicated to the 'frustrated lovers' who are willing to have mother nature, through her plants and animals, restore harmony to their sexual energy.

Love,
Howard and Nina

Foreword.

Conventional therapies normally address only the symptoms of an illness. It is clear that they are not the answer in the long run. Addressing the causes of sexual dysfunction is the first step. Nutrition is a major factor along with lifestyle, substance abuse, psychological implications and the environment. *Natural Solutions for Sexual Enhancement* is filled with many ways to build and maintain a healthy sex life.

As this book details, nutrients are unquestionably helpful for many sexual problems. A growing number of Americans are finding out what South American, Indian and Asian health practitioners have know for quite awhile; that herbs, minerals, homeopathy and vitamins all may reduce the symptoms.

Sexual dysfunction is a major cause of psychological stress, especially as people go through the hormonal changes of mid-life. Drugs, which may seem like the quick fix, only mask the true cause and do not create permanent cures. These drugs which may have harmful side effects can be substituted with natural methods that can not only alleviate the visible signs of sexual dysfunction, but may actually get to the root of the problem forever. The authors have given us a good insight into these natural alternatives. This is a timely book and one that should be read by every person, prior to embarking on drug therapies.

-Harvey Diamond, author of *Fit For Life.*

Introduction.

Sexual fulfillment can provide ultimate joy in shared intimacy, orgasm and love. It is a fable that people lose their sexuality in their later years, experience declining performance, poor responsiveness or lose their libido. Whether you are young or old, loving sex can bring with it a supreme source of mutual healing and awakening of the spirit. Sexual closeness itself can generate a healing energy, resulting in restoring intimacy and fostering a nurturing partner.

Great sex depends on good health. Most of our sexual problems stem from a poor diet, lifestyle burnout, pesticides, drugs, alcohol or a combination of all. Even if sexual problems are deemed "psychological," nutrition can be a contributing factor. The psychological problems themselves can be rooted in chemical or glandular imbalances that may be caused by poor nutrition.

Nutrition deficient, high-fat diets, overuse of drugs and alcohol, high-pressure lifestyles and low energy leads to a declining desire for sex and ultimately, no time for love. Lack of sex can also lead to lack of intimacy and a breakdown of the relationship. For single people, sexual dysfunction can prevent them from establishing lasting love and contribute to their isolation, loneliness and depression. This furthers the negative emotion that may compound the sexual dysfunctional problem.

Drugs, especially new drugs designed to increase the male erectile function, may improve psychological well being, but they will not cure the underlying problem. According to an article in Dr. Linda Page's Natural Healing Report (June 1998), "the most popular drug comes with a list of side effects. These include headaches, blurry vision and seeing blue halos after taking the drug, deadly interaction with heart medications containing nitrates, and massive heart attacks during or after sex. Men with sickle-cell anemia, leukemia or urethral inflammation run the risk of priapism (erections that last for four or more hours and can cause tissue damage and greater impotence.) Unless you have a clear medical condition, improving your libido results from a good lifestyle program, not from a pill." In *Natural Solutions for Sexual Enhancement,* we give alternatives to drug therapy. When coupled with proper nutrition, these natural solutions may in fact cure the underlying problem and eliminate the dysfunction.

Chapter 1
Sexual Problems. Why?

Common indications of sexual aging for <u>Men</u>:

Age	*Condition*
20	Semen production is at a high level.
30	Testosterone production levels out.
40	Arousal takes longer. Semen production wanes.
50	Erotic thoughts no longer sufficient for arousal. Semen further declines. Impotence increases.
60	Less sensation leading up to climax. Ejaculation diminishes.
70	Testes shrink. Several days needed between sex for recovery. Erection fades rapidly after ejaculation.

Common indications of sexual aging for <u>Women</u>:

Age	*Condition*
20	Estrogen levels are 8 to 10 times higher than in childhood.
30	Estrogen production peaks. Vaginal lubrication is at its height.
40	Arousal takes longer. With menopause approaching, the length and amount of menstrual flow begins to decrease.
50	Vaginal walls grow thinner, stiffer and drier. Estrogen levels decrease. Clitoris changes and menses ceases.
60	Estrogen production is minimal. Breasts sag.
70	Clitoris shrinks.

If nothing is done to curtail the results of aging and its associated systems breakdown, sexual dysfunction can occur. Normal aging causes a diminishing of the hormonal levels in men and women. This results in a myriad of problems, that if left unchecked can definitely alter your sex life.

Twenty million American men reportedly suffer from chronic impotence. About 25% of 65 year-old men have erectile dysfunction, and more than 50% of men over 75 report erection problems. Many men at some point in their lives will be unable to sustain an erection. This is perfectly normal and should be expected. Not all of us can be perfectly primed for sex at every moment, but when sexual dysfunction is chronic, it is time to look for a physiological explanation. In eighty five percent of the cases in which the condition persists more than a year, there is an organic reason for the problem. Erection, orgasm, and ejaculation occur under the neurological stimulus of different mechanisms. Alcohol, prostate disease, atherosclerosis, nerve damage and hormonal imbalances, (particularly those of testosterone, estrogen, and prolactin) can be an underlying cause.

We are a people of instant gratification and impatience. We tend to focus on the problem, not the cause. Therefore it is easier to go to the doctor and receive a prescription drug to get the result we desire. Unfortunately, many people rely exclusively on synthetic drugs to cure illness, speed recovery and develop a better sense of well being. All these benefits are often temporary and the drugs may elicit undesirable side effects.

Sexual dysfunction may be misdiagnosed as a psychological problem, when it may actually be caused by something physical in the body such as undiagnosed Diabetes Mellitus, a common cause of impotence in males.

Infections and anemia also can influence sexual performance. In this chapter, we describe some of the causes of sexual dysfunction. By ascertaining the reason behind the problem, you will be able to take the appropriate steps that effect a remedy.

Chemical toxicity

Most of our life styles are made up of eating processed foods, working in a toxic environment, wearing synthetic clothes, drinking alcohol, carbonated drinks and unfiltered water, while using chemical based cleaning products. The hundreds of synthetic ingredients found in our food, environment and everyday products have proven harmful to wildlife and lab animals. Now there is a new focus on whether they are putting *people* at risk by playing havoc with hormones that control reproduction and development.

Many of these hormone-disrupting chemicals origi-nate in pesticides, plastics and industrial pollutants. There have been numerous studies on why seagulls won't mate anymore. Many are considered asexual. The projected cause is an altering of their hormonal make-up due to the environmental toxins and pesticides they are ingesting with their food. Could this be filtering down to man too? Some researchers worry that toxic air pollutants and the chemical ingredients in shampoos, dyes and detergents are absorbed through the skin. Once inside the body, they may scramble our hormonal signals and reduce our desire to mate. A consequence of chemical toxicity in men is the emergence of female characteristics. In women, these toxins may contribute to infertility.

Over consumption of Alcohol

Over consumption of alcohol can affect a man's libido. It can also lead to prostate problems that may curtail sexual activity. Enlargement of the prostate may be caused by an enzyme, testosterone reductase. This interacts with testosterone and produces di-hydrotestosterone (DHT) which contributes to the decline of testosterone and also the elevation of the female hormones in men. Alcohol, especially beer, elevates levels of DHT in the body and thus can be a contributing factor in sexual dysfunction. Heavy drinkers may experience only partial erections. By eliminating the alcohol habit, the ability to have a full erection may eventually be restored.

Hormone imbalances

Sexual dysfunction caused by hormonal deficiencies is usually treated with hormone supplementation. If hormone levels in an individual are normal, augmentation won't help. In other words, testosterone supplements only increase libido and erectile function if the person already has an *insufficient* natural supply. Taking testosterone when it is not needed, may result in an enlarged prostate. Excess testosterone can also stimulate prostate cancer. Testosterone supplementation may have side effects that can include increased hair growth and abnormal liver function.

Female characteristics that appear in men may be traced to a hormone imbalance. There is an important relationship in the pituitary gland between dopamine, a neurotransmitter and the female hormone, prolactin. If dopamine levels decrease as a result of, for example, drug use, there is a corresponding increase in prolactin. Elevated levels of prolactin are associated with sexual dysfunction. Many cases of male impotency (20-25%) stem from this cause. Excess of the female hormone prolactin inhibits the production of testosterone. This can unbalance the body and contribute to the emergence of female characteristics, such as increased breast size in men. Other common symptoms are prostate problems and tender, varicose or atrophied testes.

Women experience hormonal imbalances each month during menses. Most times the only sexual dysfunctional dilemma is mood swings. Once a women reaches the menopausal years, these hormonal imbalances create definite problems with libido, vaginal dryness and painful intercourse. Many women choose to abandon their sex lives during and after menopause, much to the chagrin of their partners. Hormonal therapy may restore a woman's desire in sex and reduce many of the physical problems associated with this change of life. Use of hormones during this period should be under the direction of a health practitioner. Each woman is different and should be tested prior to undertaking hormonal therapy.

Clincal causes

Many sexual problems arise because the health of the body is being compromised somehow. For instance, the thyroid needs iodine to produce its hormones. If an iodine deficiency is present, the resulting under-active thyroid may be the root of low libido. Simply correcting the hypothyroidism may bring levels of the hormone up to par. An over-active thyroid invariably causes over-production of estrogen and all of its attendant problems for women.

Atherosclerosis (hardening of the arteries) may also occur in the penile artery. This is a common cause of impotence for almost fifty per-cent of the men over the age of 50. Factors that contribute to atherosclerosis are high cholesterol and unfavorably balanced triglyceride levels, high blood pressure, obesity, lack of exercise and smoking. When the penile artery is blocked, taking a drug to increase the blood flow to the penis may be dangerous. This is why we advise people with sexual dysfunction to find out what is causing the problem before taking a remedy with the intention of eliminating the symptom.

Infertility is becoming more prevalent and more couples are seeking answers for this problem. In addition to probable causes relating to insufficient diet and stress, there is one reason for low sperm count that is almost never considered. People with infertility problems may be cooking their sperm, rendering it inactive. In an article in the Journal of the American Medical Association on March 4, 1974, it was suggested that low sperm counts in men were caused by abnormal heat build up in their scrotums, where the sperm are produced. Since sperm can only be manufactured at temperatures slightly lower than body temperatures, excessive heat slows down or stops sperm production. High temperatures may be caused by hot showers or baths, saunas, tight fitting underwear or athletic supporters and even the use of electric blankets. Suggestions to lower scrotum temperature prior to sex include, cooler showers or baths (65°), wearing loose clothing and avoiding electric blankets.

Stress and depression can influence sex drive and performance ability. Much has been written on stress reduction including meditation, deep breathing, and attending stress reduction workshops. *You must choose what works for you.* Depression may be caused not only by psychological trauma, but because of excessive alcohol consumption, drug side-effects, food additives, nutritionally deficient diets and environmental assaults. Certain types of depression may be reduced by balancing amino acid levels, especially phenylalanine and tyrosine (found especially in meat and cheese). These amino acids are precursors of norepinephrine (the brain's version of adrenaline,) and dopamine in the brain.

Vitamin deficiencies may be a factor in sexual lubrication and inability to reach orgasm. For example, niacin causes release of histamines from the body stores. This release is necessary for achieving orgasm and also causing the sex flush or "glow" in the face, neck, etc. The niacin-caused histamine release also causes the mucous membranes of the sexual organs to secrete extra mucus needed for vaginal lubrication. Vitamin B6 aids in turning the amino acid histidine into histamine. If either vitamin B6 or niacin (vitamin B3) is deficient, the sex "machine" may not function as it was intended.

Chapter 2
Male dysfunctional problems.

Premature Ejaculation

Premature ejaculation prior to or immediately upon penetration usually has no physiological basis. In many men it is caused by being exceptionally sensitive and may occur among those who are not circumcised. Most times it is related to over-excitement or performance anxiety.

Premature ejaculation is usually resolved with specific exercises and, most important, good communication between sex partners. The most common methods recommended by sex therapists are the "squeeze" and "start/stop" techniques, which they report help in some 85 percent of cases. Both exercises involve having the partner stimulating the man's penis until he almost reaches ejaculation. Then his partner either squeezes gently the head (glans) of the penis, or simply stops, until he is able to control the urge to ejaculate.

Thinking of quick ejaculation as a disease to cure instead of a natural habit to unlearn, may have the unfortunate effect of making the situation worse. A man is never inadequate because he needs to learn new skills. He is merely untrained, and he is not a failure if he doesn't learn the new skills overnight. The herb Saw Palmetto is a natural treatment that can be used to improve male sexual performance, especially for premature ejaculation.

When treating sexual problems, Chinese medicine goes beyond the traditional approaches. Practitioners of Chinese medicine believe that vital help may be supplied by addressing energetic weakness. Yin (female energy) serves as a container for yang (male energy). If yin is weak, it may not hold the yang energy in the body resulting in the man completing the sexual process very rapidly. Chinese medicine believes that the kidneys are responsible for all sexual and reproductive functions. They determine the basic strength of our sex drive and are also in charge of gender identity. When the kidneys function well, men are more likely to feel good about themselves. When the kidneys are weak, men may feel inadequate and emasculated. Therefore, it is important to maintain the health of the kidneys through proper diet.

Lack of Erections

If you are having difficulties during lovemaking, determine whether or not you have night time erections. Healthy males have between two and five nocturnal erections, each lasting about twenty minutes. These occur during periods of REM sleep. When nocturnal erections do occur, but the men have difficulties with intercourse, chances are the problem has a psychological or emotional basis. If no erections take place, this condition may stem from organic causes that are responsible for erectile dysfunction in over 90% of men over the age of 50. An erection occurs when a message from the brain and/or spinal chord causes the muscles in the walls of the penile artery to relax. This increases the diameter of the blood vessels which allow blood to flow into the erectile tissue.

The majority of impotence or erectile inadequacy cases may be caused by the following conditions:
• When testosterone (the primary male hormone) levels are low, sexual desire may be inhibited and the ability to get an erection may be lost.
• Surgery to the pelvic area may be a contributing factor to dysfunction, as are neurological diseases such as pelvic trauma and multiple sclerosis.

• The brain directs proper blood flow to the penis to create an erection. Lack of circulation can prevent the blood from making the penis firm.

• High cholesterol is associated with impotence. For every ten point rise in cholesterol above normal, there is a 32% increase in the risk of impotence. Cholesterol can clog the penile arteries just as it does in our heart arteries. This will prevent blood from reaching the penis and thus prevent an erection. Erectile dysfunction due to atherosclerosis has been shown to be a harbinger of a heart attack or stroke.

One of the most widespread ingredients that can contribute to clogged arteries is hydrogenated or partially hydrogenated oils. Manufacturers want to extend the shelf life of oils without rancidity. To this end they process the oils which keep them in a liquid state until they reach your body. Found in margarine and as an ingredient in most store bought foodstuffs, these substances turn to sludge in the arteries. Butter and olive oil are better substitutes. If you are an avid potato chip eater, read the label. The hydrogenated oil in them may be clogging your penile artery. You can still eat potato chips but purchase health food store brands that do not contain hydrogenated oil as an ingredient.

Cholesterol imbalances also will clog arteries. Despite media reports, eating low fat diets is not the way to control cholesterol. The body needs fats, but it needs the right kind of fat. Hydrogenated oils are not healthy and low fat diets may still recommend foods that contain these oils. It is necessary that you eliminate them from your diet and read up on the advantages of essential fatty acids (EFA's). These fatty acids, Omega-6 and Omega-3 when balanced, help the body, not hurt it. They also feed the brain, which depends on fats for optimal operation. Essential fatty acids help prevent degeneration of nerves in the brain, and regulate the alpha-2-adrenergic receptors partially responsible for lack of erections in aging men. Olive oil, flax, and evening primrose oil are good choices of essential fatty acids and need to be a part of every person's diet.

If your cholesterol test is less than perfect, there is hope. Scientists are studying the interrelationship with plant sterols and sexual performance. Beta-sitosterol, found in a nutritional substance called cholestatin, blocks the intake of cholesterol by 65%. This is good news, but should not replace a proper diet. This plant sterol is also a precursor for the production of testosterone in the body.

Also, studies at the University of Bordeaux in France showed that supplementation with magnesium lowered bad cholesterol by 24% in only 10 weeks. Supplementation with magnesium should go hand in hand with pyridoxine (Vitamin B6) as it is necessary for metabolism. Chondroitin Sulfate A (CSA) also works to reduce the ability of cholesterol to adhere to artery lesions where it builds up and causes problems. As you age, the body produces less and less of CSA, therefore you may want to consider supplementation if you are at risk for atherosclerosis.

Circulatory problems originating elsewhere in the body can manifest in an inability to get or maintain an erection. Drugs that provide an extra "blood boost" are safe only if there is no clinical blockage that is preventing the circulation. Men who have heart problems or clogged arteries should weigh the risks and consider not taking drugs for impotence that speed up circulation, because penile arteries may be clogged as well. Herbs that can more naturally help circulation are Cayenne Red pepper, Ginkgo biloba, and Kava kava/Ginger root. Ginkgo biloba extract is effective due to the enhancement of blood flow through both arteries and veins without any change in systemic blood pressure.

• The brain contains nerves called alpha-2-adrenergic receptors. If these receptors are activated, they will prevent the blood valves to the penis from opening. As men age, these receptors stay activated keeping the blood from entering the penis. It is assumed this is a common function of brain deterioration as men age. This condition may be lessened by nourishing the brain with lecithin and essential fatty acids.

• Drugs use such as antihistamines, antihypertensives, antidepressants, antipsychotics, and tranquilizers can have a negative effect on penile erections.

• Endocrine disorders can add to sexual problems. When men are examined for erectile dysfunction (the new term for impotence), the doctor may conduct various blood tests to measure hormone levels. They also check various substances to make sure the thyroid and pituitary glands are functioning properly. A glucose tolerance test that helps in determining diabetes is another important key. Loss of erection is one of the first signs that tip off a doctor to Type-1 adult-onset diabetes. Your doctor may recommend further diagnostics such as an angiogram, to evaluate the arteries, and a blood test to check levels of cholesterol, triglycerides and serum lipoproteins.

A medical doctor can perform sophisticated tests to measure erections and thereby confirm normal vascular and neurological functioning. One such test is the Penile Biothesiometry method of evaluating the sensory nerves of the penis by measuring vibratory sensation with a hand-held electromagnetic device. This technique can help diagnose damaged nerves due to diabetes or alcoholism.

• As men age, their hormone levels change. Decreased male sex hormones, elevated prolactin levels and high serum estrogen levels are a factor. According to Valerie Marriott, co-author of *Growth Hormone, The Methuselah Factor,* "research has clearly demonstrated that restoring circulating levels of human growth hormone (hGH) works to not only prevent changes that normally occur with aging, but to actually reduce aging related symptoms. These include sex drive and performance. A new class of compounds, called hGH secretagogues, work by stimulating the body to release growth hormone from the pituitary so that it can restore youth and vitality. These secretagogues may contribute to acquiring and maintaining a full erection through the increased circulation that results from strengthening the heart muscles. Dr. Arnold Segredo of the Life Extension Institute notes that patients of both sexes have experienced a consistent rise in sex hormones and in sex drive with the use of this growth hormone secretagogue."

• Anxiety is a big contributor to erectile dysfunction, and performance anxiety is one of the major causes of psychologically induced impotence. Even when the root cause of impotence is physical, the situation is so emotionally charged that there are bound to be some psychological aspects involved. About eighty to ninety percent of impotence cases are physical in origin. There are, of course, instances in which men will have difficulties after emotional stress due to factors such as job loss, death of a spouse, or financial or family problems. This emotional stress may contribute to tension in the body which throws the structure out of alignment. Men report that when their pelvis was re-balanced and restructured through Craniosacral therapy, they experienced a release of tension in the lower body. These men later reported experiencing stronger and longer lasting erections, followed by more gratifying ejaculations.

A man's sexual response is an expression of his maleness, and when he cannot complete the sex act, his self-esteem is affected. This is similar to a woman's confidence being shaken when she proves to be infertile or feels undesirable. Anxiety and depression can be both the cause and effect of impotence. Depression creates something of a double-bind situation, since most antidepressant drugs are associated with impotence. Diet can be a key to overcoming depression. Although these substances can elevate your mood, several hours later the high becomes a low as your body balances out. This chemical gyrating is a cause of fatigue and depression. Avoiding stimulants such as sugar, caffeine and alcohol may in itself remove the depression.

Other contributing factors to depression are low levels of zinc, lack of sufficient quantities of amino acids, deficient levels of B vitamins and an immune system compromised through years of eating junk food. Even after a man resolves the physical source of the depression, he may experience lingering psychological effects. Impotency causes a loss of self-confidence in other areas of his life, including his social life and work. Any therapy needs to be aimed at treating the body, mind and spirit.

Low libido

Emotional symptoms leading to low libido may not be caused by mental anguish, but can be the result of dietary deficiencies and environmental assaults on the body. Those men who experience a low sex drive typically have symptoms of Vitamin B_6 (pyridoxine) deficiency, according to studies by Dr. Pat Bermond at the medical clinic of the University of Reims in France. Symptoms of this deficiency show up as cracks around the nose or mouth, a common side effect of drinking alcohol. Before you seek psychological help, you may want to analyze your lifestyle and eating habits.

Drug use, refined foods, sugar, caffeine, alcohol and tobacco all may diminish sexual desire and contribute to depression and stress. Any substance that creates a high must eventually result in a low. It's this low that affects the body and lessens the sex drive. Sexual desire originates in the brain, and it must be nourished.

A lack of healthy fats (essential fatty acids) as well as a protein deficient diet may inhibit brain activity, thus contributing to loss of sexual interest. Dietary changes may be all that is needed to restore libido. The Saw Palmetto herb can act as a mild aphrodisiac, and as a remedy for low libido. The herb, Damiana, when used in combination with other herbs, has also been used as an aphrodisiac and to improve the sexual ability of the enfeebled and aged. It is thought to work by slightly irritating the urethra, thereby producing increased sensitivity of the penis and increasing sexual desire.

Performance anxiety

At the heart of sex is an odd, almost Zen-like irony. *In order to perform our best, we must not try too hard.* We have to relax, get out of our body's way and just let it happen by itself. However, when our body is wracked with stress, tension, fatigue and anxiety and our mind is wracked with worry and distractions, sweet sex is nearly impossible. Stress and fatigue are the most common barriers to healthy sex. Stress is deadly to sex because it makes trouble on physiological, emotional and day-to-day levels. Stress also touches off a complex cascade of hormones that can have a negative effect on sex. We wind up having sex as a way of releasing stress, but when we are unable to perform, the stress increases compounding the problem. Performance anxiety creates real symptoms that diffuse sexual energy.

Performance anxiety can create a vicious circle. When we are anxious, the body puts out large amounts of norepinephrine (the brain's adrenaline), which causes vasoconstriction. In order to have an erection, a man needs to be relaxed so that the blood will flow freely into the arteries. The constriction of blood vessels due to stress works against this. Two herbs have been used in conjunction with performance anxiety: Ginseng enhances nitric oxide synthesis, regulating the muscular tone of blood vessels that control blood flow to the penis. Maca, called the Peruvian Ginseng, is another herb that is used for virility and impotency.

Although often times performance anxiety is psychologically based, diet can play a part. Stimulants such as sugar, refined foods, alcohol, caffeine and certain drugs agitate nerves in the brain, preventing relaxation. The nerves in the penis must be relaxed before they will allow the blood to create an erection. Therefore, it is important to consider the whole body if you are trying to avoid impotence. Don't blame your penis for malfunctioning. Look at what you are eating and drinking. Also consider your stress level. Worrying about an erection will be self-defeating, as the increased adrenaline secretions can agitate your nerves and prevent relaxation.

Hormonal imbalances

Men's estrogen level production goes up as their testosterone levels decrease with age. Men can experience an over estrogen condition whereby they develop higher voices, thinning hair and breast fat. An adrenal hormone that can be converted to estrogen is a contributing factor to the extra estrogen production. This occurs if the thyroid function is inadequate and the adrenals are stimulated by stress and substances such as caffeine and sugar. Over-estrogen conditions can also occur because of pesticide ingestion through foods or the environment. The body "reads" various chemical pesticides as estrogen and creates the associated over-estrogen symptoms. A man should consider clinical hormonal testing to determine his current balance, if any unusual female-like symptoms appear. Once deficiencies are determined, a course of action can be taken to rebalance the body.

Prostate problems.

The prostate is a large male gland that lies just below the neck of the bladder and around the top of the urinary tract. The primary function of the prostate is to help the semen move through the urethra during ejaculation. Because of this it enlarges during sexual arousal. If there is prolonged arousal without ejaculation, prostate pressure on the testicles becomes very uncomfortable (commonly referred to as blue balls.) Other factors can enlarge the prostate and create discomfort. Symptoms associated with enlarged prostate include frequent, painful desire to urinate, reduced flow of urine, incontinence and in extreme cases, fever, lower back pain, insomnia and fatigue. Accompanying symptoms associated with sexual dysfunction are impotence, loss of libido and possible painful ejaculation.

Obesity and hormonal changes are two well known causes of prostate enlargement. Disorders usually begin after age 35. By age 50, over 25% of all men have enlarged prostate and by age 80 the numbers grow to 80%. A diet high in saturated fats and low in the beneficial essential fatty acids puts people at the greatest risk. Factored in as causes are hormonal imbalances, low fiber diets, spicy foods, and excessive use of alcohol and caffeine, eating meat from animals injected with hormones, prostaglandin depletion, an exhausted lymph system from chronic usage of antihistamines, a lack of exercise, zinc deficiency and venereal disease.

Enlargement of the prostate may be caused by an enzyme, testosterone reductase, which interacts with testosterone and produces di-hydrotestosterone (DHT). Alcohol, especially beer, elevates levels of DHT in the body and thus can be a contributing factor. The herb, Saw Palmetto supports prostate health by promoting a reduction in DHT in tissue by over 40%. It balances the body's hormones to block painful prostate enlargement, and can be an effective natural treatment. Pygeum africanum, an herb, also lowers DHT levels by blocking cholesterol production.

Vasectomies also lie suspect in contributing to prostate problems. Science has long debated whether risk of prostate cancer is a result of vasectomy (the contraceptive procedure which severs or seals off the vessel that carries sperm from the testes.) New studies on two large group of men show that vasectomies increase risk of prostate cancer. In one study of 73,000 men between 1986 and 1990, those with vasectomies had a 66% greater risk of prostate cancer. In a separate study, vasectomies increased the risk of prostate cancer by 56%. After a vasectomy, sperm build up in the sealed off vas deferens. The body re-absorbs these cells which confuses the immune system, making it less alert to tumor cells. It also causes the body's defenses to mount a response against its own tissue. In addition, a vasectomy affects hormone secretions in the testes and lowers prostatic fluid. When the natural movement of sperm and hormones are artificially prevented, numerous health problems may arise.

Men who have chronic constipation may create prostate problems. In a healthy person there is space between the colon and the prostate. Constipation causes the colon to swell and push against the prostate. If this condition is chronic, bacteria from the colon can migrate through the muscles and mucous membranes of the colon and penetrate the stroma tissue surrounding the prostate. This condition is called prostatitis. Kenneth Yasny PhD, in his book *Put Hemorrhoids and Constipation Behind You* gives suggestions that may alleviate constipation. Eat moist foods and drink lots of water to help waste move through our system. Eat high fiber foods that absorb moisture, and grease your intestines with polyunsaturated or monounsaturated oils.

Unfortunately, a cardinal rule in natural prostate recovery is abstinence. Sexual intercourse irritates the prostate and delays the repair process. Treating prostate problems with drug therapy comes with a list of side effects that can include loss of libido and decreased potency. To naturally reduce inflammation of the prostate you should avoid alcohol, caffeine, carbonated drinks, tomato juice, fried and refined foods and red meat. A deficiency in zinc may lead to changes in the size, structure and function of the prostate. Because of its very high zinc content, Bee pollen can have great value in healing the prostate gland when used as supplement.

A specialty diet is included in Linda Rector Page's *Healthy Healing* book that includes high fiber, whole grains, low fats and a cleansing with lemon juice and water. She mentions many herbal treatments. These include Saw palmetto (prevents the breakdown of testosterone to DHT), Echinacea/goldenseal (for inflammation), White oak (to shrink swollen prostate), Nettles (relieves frequent urination), Hydrangea (reduce sediment), Garlic (an anti-ineffective), and Damiana (wards off infection).

Spirituality

A sexually whole man needs to be in touch with his own vulnerability and must recognize feelings that tend to block intimacy. To be close to a woman he must first develop trust and intimacy with himself. This usually means some soul-searching and/or therapy and support groups.

James Green, in his book, *The Male Herbal* writes that the number-one killer of men is broken hearts. Heart disease is the primary killer of American males, so his metaphor is appropriate. The inability to express emotions or show vulnerability contributes to stress, a leading cause of heart disease as well as sexual dysfunction. When we connect with our inner selves, all facets of our nature can be expressed. To the extent that men can do that, they will earn the sexual intimacy they want and deserve.

Chapter 3
Female dysfunctional problems.

Women have a natural advantage over men when it comes to understanding their own bodies. Their biology is more complicated, with menstrual cycles and pregnancy compelling them to seek information about their physiology. Women are also more apt to seek help for problems, either from one another or from a professional source.

Not having to worry about performance anxiety, the woman can engage in the sex act whether she is interested or not. Vaginal lubricants can substitute for her lack of libido, and those who are gifted actresses can fool even the most scrutinizing partner into thinking they have reached an orgasm. Unfortunately, for women who really want to enjoy sex but are facing sexual dysfunction, they are normally told to seek psychological help. Although looking at the root of sexual hang-ups may help in reducing anxiety, and increasing orgasmic ability, it doesn't do much for vaginal dryness, loss of libido, menopausal conditions, infertility and vaginal atrophy.

Many of these conditions can be helped by taking natural progesterone or natural estrogen (estriol). When using the natural progesterone, you must ask questions of the manufacturer. Natural progesterone is not the same as synthetic progestins which have side effects such as depression, acne, and weight gain. Synthetic progestins may be carcinogenic and inhibit the production of your own natural progesterone. Natural progesterone actually stimulates its own synthesis in the body. Semi-synthetic progesterone if used as an isolate is known as Progesterone U.S.P. Although it is extracted from wild yams, it may not include some of the plant's natural enzymes, peptides or other phytosterols having been destroyed in the extraction process. These are important phytochemicals the body needs to nurture itself. Semi-synthetic progesterone may be quite effective in reducing menopausal symptoms at the onset, but it may have undesirable long term side effects. Even a small dosage of 25mg/day can block pathways in the endocrine system, raising cholesterol levels and requiring stronger and stronger dosages to work as it will eventually desensitize receptor sites.

Progesterone replacement is best accomplished by using a product containing Progesterone USP along with wild yam (Dioscorea) whole plant extracts, which have a modulating or balancing effect on how the body utilizes the progesterone isolate. The resultant product is nearly identical to the progesterone that the body produces. The method of extraction must be one that leaves all the nutrients in tact. James Jamieson, pharmacologist, is currently working with over 110 species of wild yams. He says, "You have to be careful not to disturb the delicate synergism and balance as each phytogen, peptide, enzyme, co-enzyme as well as other co-factors because they all have different and remarkable actions and activities in the body."

Synthetic, semi-synthetic and many "natural" progester-ones do not respect mother nature's wisdom and will provide only that substance that gets immediate results. Also, many wild yam creams or tinctures can be hazardous to your health because they contain pesticides, whose residue will mimic pseudoestrogens and definitely destroy the endocrine balance. Be sure that your wild yam supplement of choice is organic and has all its natural nutrients in tact.

Addressing a female sexual dysfunction does not mean going out and indiscriminately purchasing supple-ments based on media hype. It is essential that you determine your hormonal deficiencies through tests conducted by your gynecologist or health practitioner. You can then decide on a course of action.

Stress and loss of libido

Many factors affect a loss of sexual desire. Women are greatly influenced by their emotions and their menstrual cycles. Emotions affect hormone levels and the endocrine system. When stress, anxiety, depression or anger festers inside our heads, the body reacts in fatigue, pain, and loss of libido. If we want to permanently fix the problem, we must address the cause of the change in sexual interest rather than just take an aphrodisiac.

Many times the emotional symptoms are not caused by mental anguish, but can be the result of dietary deficiencies and environmental assaults on the body. Before you seek psychological help, you may want to analyze your lifestyle and eating habits. By eliminating aggravants, you may change the physiology of the mental condition. Foods that have been processed can compromise the immune system and play havoc with your sex drive. Sugar, alcohol and caffeine although may momentarily give you a high, they eventually drain the body, creating many symptoms including fatigue and depression. Excess amounts of wheat and white flour also can contribute to low libido.

Since the brain originates sexual desire, it must be nourished. Dietary changes may be all that is needed to restore libido. A lack of essential fatty acids, as well as a protein deficient diet, may inhibit neural stimulation, thus contributing to sexual apathy. The Saw palmetto herb and Damania herb when taken as a supplement, may act as mild aphrodisiacs and as a remedy for low libido.

Craniosacral Therapy may also help lack of libido by adjusting the body. Tension and stress are thereby released, allowing the nerves to relax and become more sexually sensitive. Supplementing with DHEA (a hormone naturally produced by the adrenal glands) may increase libido in some women. As we age, the body's production of DHEA gradually decreases. According to Beth M. Ley in her book *DHEA: Unlocking the Secrets to the Fountain of Youth*, she notes that studies indicated supplemental DHEA can improve sex drive and increase fertility.

Menopause

Menopause is the time of life when a woman's ovaries stop producing eggs, and the hormonal secretions that orchestrate menstruation diminish. There is also a decline in vaginal wetness during sexual arousal, decreased vaginal elasticity, loss of interest in sex, lack of increase in breast size during sexual stimulation and fewer and sometimes painful contractions of the uterus during orgasm. Nearly all of these changes can be explained by hormonal imbalances.

During menopause, the tissues of the bladder and urethra also may become more sensitive. This may increase the frequency of urination, with some women needing to void several times during the night or during sex. A full bladder will definitely curtail a woman's interest in intercourse. It can also result in increased urinary tract infections, urinary burning, and leaking of urine upon coughing, laughing or sneezing. Women who experience yeast infections, urinary problems or even constipation, can lose interest in sex because intercourse becomes uncomfortable.

Establishing adequate hormonal levels can reduce many of these symptoms. As stated previously, supplementation may also be the key to youth. Vitamin B complex supports the nervous system, reducing anxiety and stress. Calcium decreases emotional irritability and magnesium relieves mood swings. Bioflavonoids help to regulate estrogen levels and many herbs may be just what the 'doctor' ordered for a variety of sexual maladies. CranioSacral therapies may help with menopausal symptoms by readjusting and rebalancing the body. Women do not have to worry about erections or staying power, but in order to have intercourse, they must correct vaginal atrophy and dryness.

Vaginal Dryness

Difficulties having intercourse can be compounded if a woman's vagina is not lubricated. Vaginal dryness can appear as itching and burning which may occur throughout the day. This uncomfortable condition may make a woman unwilling to even consider having sex. Creams and lotions may be temporary fixes, but are not long term cures. Women in the menopausal years are more prone to vaginal dryness, but it can occur at any age.

Birth control pills may have a side effect that manifests as vaginal dryness. Dietary deficiencies such as zinc, vitamins A, C and E and an improper balance of essential fatty acids can contribute to this condition. Menopause creates a hormone imbalance. The lack of normal levels of estrogen can cause the vaginal walls to lose their elasticity and become somewhat drier and thinner. Vaginal secretions become less acidic, and there is more risk of vaginal infections. The mucous secretions from the cervix also decrease, and the vagina itself shrinks, becoming shorter and narrower. These changes are noticeable during intercourse and lead women to wonder whether the days of sexual pleasure are over.

Treating this condition with dietary supplementation of zinc, vitamins A, C and E and a good essential fatty acid source such as flax, will help to support the mucous membranes and relieve the drying of the vaginal lining. Applying a progesterone cream to the vaginal lips may also solve the problem. Adding a growth hormone (hGH), secretagogue to your list of supplements may also cure vaginal dryness as well as increase libido. In the book, *Growth Hormone: Reversing Human Aging Naturally*, Dr. L.E. Dorman points out that hGH secretagogues, work by stimulating the body to release growth hormone from the pituitary so that it can restore youth and vitality. It's effects include increased vaginal lubrication and improvement in libido. This is a natural way to help the body remember what it used to do and do it again, regardless of age.

Vaginal atrophy

Many women experience a closing down of the vagina during or after menopause. This alone would deter the interest in intercourse which could be very painful. Many times this problem is caused by an imbalance in progesterone vs. estrogen levels and also can traced to a diminishing level of testosterone in the female body. It is best to consult a health practitioner who specializes in gynecology, and request a hormone test to see where your levels are.

Using natural progesterone cream and supplements containing testosterone may reduce the atrophy and return the vagina to a more elastic condition. Testosterone levels decline in a woman starting at age 40. By age 60 many women have lost up to 60% of their ability to release testosterone. Surgical procedures such as removing the ovaries can also affect testosterone production. In addition to vaginal atrophy, lack of testosterone can cause loss of sexual desire, decreased sensitivity to sexual stimulation and diminished capacity for orgasm. Testosterone is an androgenic hormone produced by the adrenals and the ovaries and is necessary to produce a sex drive. Supplementation with plant derived compounds that support physiologic functions associated with testosterone may be necessary. Ginseng, an herbal source of plant testosterone has also been shown to stimulate production of testosterone in the body. If this procedure doesn't help, you may need to apply an estriol (natural estrogen) cream.

Hormonal Imbalance

Hormonal imbalances can be caused by various reasons and create unpleasant side effects that reduce sexual interest. Excess estrogen is associated with heart problems, stroke and hypoxia (lack of oxygen). Women who have ratios of less than five progesterone to one estrogen, are prone to cyclic seizures, excessive bleeding, fibrocystic breast disease, and ovarian cysts. An over abundance of estrogen also promotes thyroid deficiencies because it inhibits thyroid secretion. This results in symptoms such as headaches, frequent infections, insomnia, fatigue, depression, constipation and cancer to name a few.

You may be getting excess estrogen through your food and the environment. Many chemicals like chlorine, pesticides and PCBs (petroleum byproducts) mimic estrogen in the body, creating mixed messages. The brain compensates for this excess "estrogen" and creates symptoms that are akin to those for actual hormonal imbalances. This is basically what is happening in the bird communities, altering their desire to mate.

The ovaries aren't the only producers of estrogen. Androgens (specifically androstenedione, an adrenal hormone) can be converted to estrogen in both men and women. In women, after menopause, the conversion of androgens and progesterone to estrogen can occur if thyroid function is inadequate and the adrenals are stimulated by substances that include sugar and caffeine. Adrenal exhaustion can also be caused by the stressful and hectic lifestyles we lead. The result is that this hormonal imbalance causes a masculinizing effect on women by changing the shape of their body and growing facial hair.

When taking supplemental hormones, choose brands that include a healthy ratio of (10) progesterone to (1) estrogen. Unless it balances by progesterone, estrogen may increase the growth of existing cancers especially when it is taken in continuous small doses. It can create other side effects as well, including increased risk of pituitary cancers, liver dysfunction, gall bladder attacks, water retention, and weight gain.

Many herbs can assist in balancing the hormones. Dong Quai is a bittersweet herb that is widely used in the Orient as a tonic for the female reproductive system. Dong Quai has a regulating and normalizing effect on hormone production. Maca, Licorice, Wild yam, Chaste Tree berry and Black Cohosh are other herbs that may be considered support for hormone functions.

Spiritual energy

Many women still suffer from the mistaken idea that spiritual energy and sexual energy are opposing forces. Women sometimes deny their sexuality in order to be more spiritual, creating a tremendous conflict within themselves, and eventually blocking the very energy they are seeking. Actually, spiritual energy and sexual energy are simply ways of expressing love for themselves and others. Both are very powerful, and women need to honor their sexual energy as a spiritual force.

Chapter 4
Natural solutions for men and women.

We have touched on several natural treatments for sexual dysfunction in the previous chapters. Since there are different solutions for individual conditions, we have made a chart to help you choose the right treatment. Each item is explained later in this chapter. Please refer to it for your specific needs.

FOR MEN

	Prostate	Premature ejaculation	Erectile dysfunction	Performance anxiety	Hormone imbalance
Aloe			x		
Aromatherapy				x	
Bee pollen	x		x	x	x
Bioflavonoids	x	x	x		x
Craniosacral			x	x	
EFAs	x		x	x	x
Electrolytes	x	x	x	x	x
Enzymes	x	x	x		x
hGH	x		x	x	x
Lecithin	x	x	x	x	x
Nutritional yeast	x		x	x	x
Royal jelly			x		
Sea vegetables	x		x	x	x
Velvet antler	x		x	x	x
Wheat grass	x		x	x	x
Homeopathic					
Agnus	x		x		
Cantharis			x	x	
Sabel	x		x		

For Men (continued)

	Prostate	Premature ejaculation	Erectile dysfunction	Performance anxiety	Hormone Imbalance
Minerals:					
Chromium	x		x		x
Calcium	x	x		x	
Iodine	x			x	
Iron				x	
Magnesium	x	x		x	
Manganese					x
Phosphorus				x	
Potassium	x			x	x
Selenium	x			x	x
Zinc	x		x		x
Herbs:					
Ashwaganda			x		
Cayenne			x		
Chaste berry			x		
Damiana	x		x		
Garlic			x	x	x
Gingko biloba			x		
Ginseng	x		x	x	
Kava kava				x	
Licorice			x		
Maca	x		x	x	x
Muira puma			x		
Pygeum	x		x		
Sarsaparilla			x		
Saw palmetto	x		x		
Similax	x		x		
Tribulus					x
Valerian		x		x	
Yohimbe	x		x	x	x
Vitamins					
Vitamin A	x		x		x
Vitamin B5, B6			x	x	
Vitamin E & C	x		x		x

FOR WOMEN

	Low Libido	Menopause	Vaginal Dryness	Vaginal Atrophy	Hormone Imbalance
Aloe		x			
Aromatherapy	x				
Bee pollen	x	x			x
Bioflavonoids	x	x	x	x	x
Craniosacral therapy		x			
EFAs	x	x	x	x	x
Electrolytes	x	x	x	x	x
Enzymes	x	x			x
fermented Soy	x	x			x
hGH	x	x			x
Lecithin	x	x	x	x	x
Royal jelly	x	x			x
Sea vegetables	x				
Velvet antler	x	x			x
Nutritional yeast	x	x			x
Wheat grass	x				
Homeopathic					
Agnus	x				
Cantharis	x	x			
Sabal	x				
Minerals					
Calcium	x	x			x
Chromium	x	x			x
Iodine	x	x			
Iron	x	x			
Magnesium	x	x			x
Manganese	x				
Phosphorus	x				
Potassium	x				
Selenium		x			x
Zinc	x	x			x

For women (continued)

	Low libido	Menopause	Vaginal Dryness	Vaginal Atrophy	Hormone Imbalance
Herbs					
Ashwaganda	x				
Avena sativa	x				
Black Cohosh	x	x			x
Chaste Tree berry	x	x			x
Damiana	x				
Dendrobium leaf	x				x
Dong Quai	x	x			x
Ginseng	x	x			x
Kava kava & Ginger	x				
Licorice root	x				x
Maca	x	x		x	x
Muira puama	x				
Sarsaparilla		x			x
Tribulus	x				x
Yohimbe	x				
Wild yam		x			x
Vitamins					
Vitamin A	x		x	x	x
Vitamin B3	x				
Vitamin B5, B6	x				
Vitamin B12	x	x			x
Vitamin E	x	x	x	x	x

Natural solutions

Aloe Vera juice is an excellent source of polysaccharides. Polysaccharides are probably less well known to most of us than vitamins, minerals, or even fatty acids. They are natural substances made of proteins and sugars. Together with collagen, they form the glue that holds together all our body tissues and give strength and elasticity to tissues and membranes. Among their other functions, they boost the production of seminal fluid and increase potency and sex drive.

Aromatherapy is based on the fact that the fastest way to alter a mood state is with smell. The information from scents is directly relayed to the hypothalamus, where motivation, moods and creativity all begin. The aromatherapy essential oils work through hormone-like neurochemicals to produce their sensations. When the scent of an essential oil enters through the nose, it stimulates a sensory cell that sends a message to the limbic system (the emotional brain). This system controls emotion and triggers memory and sexual response.

Sexuality-enhancing aromatherapy oils for men include: Basil, Cedarwood, Jasmine, Lavender, Patchouli, Sandalwood and Ylang Ylang.

Oils especially nice for women are: Clary Sage, Cypress, Geranium, Jasmine, Lavender, Neroli, Rose and Ylang Ylang.

Many of these essential oils are interchangeable for men and women. Smell is a potent "good medicine" that is highly individual. The best ways to use essential oils are:

  a. Inhalations straight from the bottle and/or a
     diffuser in the bedroom.
  b. Bathe either by yourself and/or with a partner.
  c, Massage either yourself and/or a partner.

Note: It is important to use pure, high-grade essential oils for best result. They need to be blended with a base oil for skin application.

Bee pollen called the only nutritionally complete food, is well known as a sexual system vitalizer, for both men and women. Bee pollen is the key to prostate health. Its high concentration of zinc is important in boosting zinc levels of the prostate and semen. It also contains magnesium which is needed to create prostaglandins or hormones which have an energizing activity upon the prostate. Its many nutrients include lecithin and essential fatty acids, both needed by the brain, nerves and sexual system. It also contains natural plant steroids thought to nourish and stimulate the glands that produce our sex hormones. Bee pollen may improve our general and sexual condition, which will have a significant effect on performance, and improved sperm production.

CranioSacral Therapy. John Upledger,, D.O., O.M.M. reported on this effective therapy. He has given us the following information on the success of this therapy. Although there have been no formal controlled scientific studies of the effects of CranioSacral Therapy (CST) upon sexual function of any kind, there are an abundance of case reports and clinical observations that suggest that CST is efficacious in the treatment of a rather wide variety of sexual dysfunctions. These range from male impotency and female orgasmic failure to menstrual disorders, menopausal syndromes and infertility.

Usually where CST is effective, the causal factors in these sexual dysfunctions can be traced to problems with the nervous system, the endocrine system, the blood vascular system, and stasis of body fluids, especially in the pelvis. They also stem from structural problems of the body pelvis and/or the lower spine and the related muscles, tendons, ligaments, etc. as well as with the craniosacral system.

Good sexual function requires a fairly well tuned and coordinated function of all of the aforementioned system and structures, as well as the organs directly involved. CST is a soft-touch technique approach that enhances the body's own inherent self-corrective processes. The most powerful effects of CST are upon the craniosacral system itself, through which a balance in the total nervous system is often achieved. The effects of this rebalancing include stress reduction, relaxation enhancement, reduction of spasm and hypertonus in tissues all over the body, as well as enhanced fluid exchange at all levels, from blood vascular to the flow of fluids across cell membranes.

CST also assists glandular function directly by its favorable influences upon the pituitary and pineal gland which, in turn, serve to regulate the remainder of the endocrine glands throughout the body. Secondarily, CST enhances the effect of all these glands by improving the movement of the fluids throughout the body as these fluids carry the hormones secreted by these glands. Also, these bodily fluids are the transportation method which serves the newly discovered peptide system. This involves a wide array of protein substances, many of which are produced by the nervous system, and have marked effects upon the function of all organs and tissues involved in both male and female sexual functions.

Quite often patients are treated by CST for other problems, such as low back pain or headaches. During the course of treatment, the patient will frequently confide that there is a noticeable improvement in sexual function, be it heightened interest, a more gratifying sexual experience or a reduction of PMS and/or menopausal symptoms. It is quite often that male patients, as their pelvic structures are rebalanced and released from tension, experience significantly stronger and longer lasting erections and more gratifying ejaculations, thereby reducing their performance anxiety.

Female infertility is a chief concern for many patients. Quite often a loosening and rebalancing of the pelvic structures and tissues is all that is required for conception to occur. If fertility treatments have been unsuccessfully undertaken prior to CST, a multiple birth may be facilitated. If this is a concern it may be advisable to stop the use of fertility drugs about four to six months before beginning CST. Since CranioSacral Therapy is virtually risk-free and is economical, it is probably worth a try for any kind of sexual dysfunction because they are often related to physiological and/or structural problems effectively treated by CST.

Enzymes. Enzymes are essential in maintaining internal cleanliness, health, youth and strength. Since digestive enzymes are only found in raw foods, our pancreas must produce enzymes when we eat cooked foods. Americans eat more cooked food than raw which causes their pancreas to work overtime and grow in size resulting in pancreatic illness. Digestive disorders, arthritis, sexual dysfunction and short term memory loss are associated with enzyme deficiencies. Enzyme deficiencies mean that undigested food in the intestinal tract may give a home to bacteria and parasites. In addition, if digestion is not functioning properly, then protein won't be broken down into free form amino acids needed by neurotransmitters in the brain, which control our sexual drive and responses.

To reduce the extra work of the pancreas and to conserve our supply of body enzymes, we can supplement our diet with plant enzymes every time we eat cooked or processed food. This type of enzyme works throughout the digestive tract, whereas some types just work in the stomach. Benefits include less stomach and intestinal diseases as well as prevention of impotency, which some have referred to as an enzyme deficiency disease

Essential Fatty Acids and Prostaglandins. A high fat diet will actually decrease sexuality. Men who eat a high-fat meal will have an immediate 25% drop in their testosterone levels and women will tend to feel sleepy. Improper balance of fats may create a high level of LDL cholesterol that reduces the ability of the penis to receive 'erection signals' from the brain. When the arteries are clogged due to a high-fat diet, penis tissue flexibility is reduced, which results in the shortening and weakening of erections.

No fat or low fat diets are not the answer. The body and the brain needs fats, but not the kind found in most junk foods. Olive oil and butter keep a liquid consistency once the enter the body. Hydrogenated or partially hydrogenated oils (found in snack foods, most commercial cooking oils and as ingredients in other packaged foods) turn to sludge in the body and tend to stick to lesions in arterial walls. This sludge eventually builds up and clogs the artery. If the brain is fat deficient, proper signals will not be sent to the sexual organs and performance will be compromised.

Essential fatty acids (EFA's) are needed by the brain, the nervous system, the immune system, the skin, the glands and all the vital organs. In other words, they are necessary to every cell in our body. In addition, they protect the cells from viruses and bacteria. They are the precursors of hormone-like substances called prosta-glandins, which are important for sexual response. The two essential fatty acids that we need to get from our diet are alpha linolecic acid (Omega 3 group) and linolenic (Omega 6 group). CLA (conjugated linoleic acid) belongs to the family of omega-6 fatty acids. CLA may increase production of prostaglandin E1, that increases brain levels of the hormone somatotropin. This hormone increases growth output that, in turn, increases testosterone.

Essential Fatty Acids (EFA'S) help provide moisture and softness to the skin, vagina and bladder (especially important when estrogen level decreases). Low EFA'S cause some women to experience cramping. Men may experience insufficient ejaculate during intercourse. Both sexes may become infertile because of EFA deficiencies. Essential fatty acids increase energy levels, especially physical activity. We are tired less quickly, recover faster, feel more like being sexually active and stay alert later in the evening. An excellent source of EFA's is Flax seed (also known as horny food). You can find flax supplements in capsules or as a primary ingredient in certain snack food bars. Flax also can be purchase in the raw seed form to grind in your coffee grinder or pre-ground ready to use on cereal, salads or in health drinks.

Green Foods.
• *Chlorella* increases the efficiency of our immune system to protect us from viruses, bacteria, cancer cells and stress. It's chlorophyll is very effective against bacteria and may be more effective than vitamin A, C or E as an antioxidant which can guard against urinary infections, yeast infections in women, prostate illness and other maladies that would deter sexual interest.
• *Sea vegetables* such as kelp, spirulina and blue green algae, provide a high source of micronutrients.

Kelp sparks vital enzyme reactions in the body and supports the thyroid.

Hawaiian spirulina is considered one of the premium green superfoods. It is a concentrated whole food source of phyto-nutrients, supplying a rich mixture of enzymes, chlorophyll and complete vegetarian protein.

Blue green algae is nutrient dense. Small doses may provide biologically active vitamins, minerals, trace minerals, amino acids, simple carbohydrates, enzymes, fatty acids and chlorophyll. Its protein content is of a type that may be more easily broken down and assimilated by the body, than the protein in meats.

• *Wheat grass* is an excellent source of protein and essential fatty acids. It is rich in enzymes, B-complex vitamins and vitamin C. Wheat grass is high in fiber and minerals with significant amounts of calcium, iron and zinc. Viktoras Kulvinskas in his book, *The Lover's Diet*, says that wheat grass is the highest vibrational food on the planet. Science shows that the chlorophyll of wheat grass is nearly like the hemoglobin of human blood. People who eat wheat grass have reported an increase in stamina. It may help increase sexual desire for both men and women, especially when combined with blue-green algae.

Lecithin is a fat-like substance normally produced in the liver. Nutrients enter and leave our cells via cell membranes mostly composed of lecithin. If it is in short supply, this membrane will harden and nutrients will be kept out. The best thing lecithin does is to dissolve the bad cholesterol in the blood and help additionally to open capillaries and blood vessels. Combining lecithin and crystalloid electrolytes will slowly rebalance and eliminate the problem of penile dysfunction. Lecithin is an important constituent of both vaginal and seminal fluids. It also affects the sex center of the brain, the transmission of nerve messages for sexuality and the endocrine glands

Minerals. All of us, men and women alike, are made up of organic elements, primarily oxygen, carbon, hydrogen, nitrogen and inorganic minerals such as calcium and potassium. We can tolerate a deficiency of vitamins longer than a deficiency of minerals. A slight change in the cellular level of important minerals may endanger health and survival.

While it is true, that both sexes can feel the effects of mineral deficiencies, it is also true that women are more likely to be deficient. The stress reactions triggered during menopause, deplete minerals. Stress affects body chemistry and depletes minerals. Trace minerals (electrolytes) are involved in the health of the glands and the production of the hormones that control the use of calcium in the body. Because of this, they need to be one of the first supplements taken for the prevention of menopausal symptoms, and also to reduce the risk of osteoporosis.

In men, one of the main physical causes of impotence is atherosclerosis of the penile arteries, which restricts blood flow. This can be traced back to mineral imbalance. It is thought that in a significant number of men hardening of the arteries is caused by a diet too high in certain fats and sugars. What is not considered, is that this problem may be caused by a lack of trace minerals including chromium and manganese.

Narrowed blood vessels restrict blood flow and limit erection. It is well known fact that the minor capillaries and blood vessels, which are similar in both the brain and the penis structure, have two major factors that work against constant blood flow. Proper circulation is absolutely necessary for the penis to get and maintain an erection. As they age, many men face a breakdown in brain function. If not arrested, this can cause senility or Alzheimer's. Many times this condition stems from too much aluminum in the body.

We can ingest this metal from deodorant, cookware, antacids and baking powder. Further, when there is a drop in the trace element levels in the body, this problem is compounded. Erectile dysfunction may actually be a harbinger for physical problems originating in the brain

How does one go about reversing terrible ailments such as erectile dysfunction and senility? The first step is to restore the body's mineral balance as nature intended. This part of the healing process involves restoring the body's proper pH (acid-alkaline balance). Re-establishment of pH can be achieved with a proper mineral solution. In this case, liquid crystalloid electrolytes can be very effective. The body will slowly rebalance and eliminate the penile dysfunction.

Over time, electrolyte supplementation can break down mineral deposits wherever they are in the body. Arthritic conditions, urinary gravel and kidney stones may be reduced. Restoring the body to a healthy energetic state enhances sexual desire and performance. Trace minerals (electrolytes) are called the "spark plugs" for sexual energy for both men and women. For further information on crystalloid electrolyte minerals, you can refer to the booklet, *Crystalloid Electrolytes, Our body's energy source for the new millennium* listed on the last page of this book.

The essential trace minerals needed by the body include boron, manganese, copper, iodine, zinc, cobalt, chromium and selenium. Taking too much of one essential mineral may upset the balance and function of other minerals. For instance, excess zinc can interfere with calcium absorption and vice versa. More is not necessarily better when it comes to minerals. Many supplements cram scores of minerals into their product, but the body works best with just the basics. Following are minerals that have a particular relevance to sexuality.

• *Calcium* is essential for strong bones, teeth and muscles. Concern over calcium deficiency has come to the forefront due to the problem of osteoporosis in post-menopausal women. Most women have diets low in calcium and require supplements long before menopause. Calcium needs to be taken with magnesium and vitamin D or it will not be properly utilized by the body. The ratio usually is 1:1 and these minerals are normally taken at bed time where they are easily absorbed. When taken with magnesium, calcium acts as a natural relaxant to assist in treating performance anxiety.

• *Chromium*, acting with insulin, is required for glucose utilization. It is an essential nutrient required for anyone with low blood sugar that may create mood swings which will alter sex drive and libido. Deficiency in chromium has been known to detrimentally affect cholesterol levels, contribute to heart trouble, diabetes and hypoglycemia.

• *Iron* is an extremely important mineral for the development of healthy red blood cells since it is the central element in hemoglobin, which carries oxygen to the tissues. Menstruating and pregnant women have increased requirement for iron. Although both iron deficiency and iron overload can be dangerous, iron is necessary for metabolic health. It can nourish an under-active thyroid to trigger increases in libido. (The thyroid secretions released into the bloodstream determine our body's basic energy level and also affect the rate at which sex hormones are created.)

• *Iodine* is an essential mineral for the functioning of the thyroid gland and is an integral part of thyroxin. (Thyroxin is one of the master hormones that require metabolic functioning. It promotes growth, stimulates cholesterol synthesis and regulates other glandular functions.) Low levels of iodine can result in a sluggish thyroid and can even lead to hypothyroidism and goiters. Women with under or overactive thyroid glands are likely to have irregular periods or severe PMS symptoms.

• *Manganese* is a trace mineral important for the activation of many enzyme systems in our body. It is also involved in female sex hormone production. Manganese strengthens the reproductive system and is important in the function of the mammary glands.

• *Magnesium* contributes to the production of sex hormones. Women suffering symptoms of PMS or menstrual cramps may find some relief from taking a magnesium supplement, as it increases progesterone levels. This mineral is also beneficial for counteracting depression. When combined with calcium, magnesium acts as a natural relaxant which may help reduce stress associated with performance anxiety.

• *Phosphorus* is essential to support brain and nerve activity. When taken with calcium and magnesium it helps maintain sexual desire. It is important in energy production and aides in absorption of other vitamins and herbs. Phosphorus increases muscle performance while decreasing muscle fatigue important for stamina in men.

• *Potassium* is a specific mineral for men trying to conceive. It strengthens the heart and circulation, and combats fatigue. This is especially important for male virility and conception, since potassium controls hypertension, depression and stress.

• *Selenium* is an important micronutrient often lacking in the average diet. Requirements for men are higher than for women. There is a high concentration of the mineral in semen, therefore selenium is needed for sperm production. It works together with vitamin E to reduce free-radical damage, and it protects the immune system and the heart. It Also helps women promote progesterone.

• *Zinc* is of major importance in the male reproductive system. In fact, one of the highest concentrations of this mineral is found in the prostate. However, zinc is important throughout the body and is absolutely vital for the function of many enzyme systems. One of zinc's many roles is in the stimulation of the male hormone, testosterone. This hormone assists in men's capacity to develop an erection and to ejaculate. Infertility and loss of sex drive may be the result of a zinc deficiency. In women, a deficiency may cause disruption of menstruation, reduced vaginal lubrication and loss of sexual interest.

Nutritional yeast is an excellent source of protein that contains Vitamin B complex and amino acids. Amino acids have proven to be important for men addressing infertility problems. The following amino acids are useful in treating sexual dysfunction:

L-Arginine may help increase sperm production and motility besides being the well-known boost for the hormone testosterone.

L-Carnitine has shown general improvement in circulation and metabolism and increased sperm count.

Tyrosine boosts dopamine levels (associated with memory ability, sense of well-being and with sex drive).

Phenylalanine is one of the essential amino acids that is a precursor of the neurotransmitter epinephrin, norepinephrine and dopamine, all of which are influential in sexual arousal and response and relieving depression.

Tryptophan is a precursor of serotonin, the body's stress reducer.

Royal jelly contains hormone-like substances that support the glands and reproductive system. It is the only natural source of pure acetylcholine, a very important compound involved in the conduction of nerve and sexual impulses. Sperm count and mobility increases, and frequency of ejaculation also increases.

Soy is rich in phytoestrogens (plant estrogens) called isoflavones. These isoflavones resemble the human sex hormone estrogen. Research indicates that soybeans and their potent phytoestrogens may help alleviate some of the symptoms of menopause that may interfere with sexual desire. The most common form of soy is unfermented which means the soybean hasn't begun to sprout. In the infant stage soybeans produce enzyme inhibitors. Ingesting them results in gastric distress, reduced protein digestion and chronic deficiencies in amino acid uptake. Since one of the benefits of soy is plant based protein and calcium, if you are unable to digest it, these benefits disappear. Most of the soy milk, tofu and soy protein drinks are made with unfermented soy. In fermented (or sprouted) soy which is harvested after the bean has started to sprout, more of the enzyme inhibitors are deactivated therefore are much more digestible. This type of soy can be found in foods such as tempe, miso and sprouted soy powder supplements.

Velvet antlers, when harvested (by a method that doesn't hurt the elk/deer) at a certain time of the year, becomes a very potent source of hormones, minerals, amino acids and enzymes as well as cartilage. Elk and deer in their natural setting eat a variety of herbs, including ginseng, which is considered an aphrodisiac.

Velvet antlers contain both the male and female hormone precursors. One of the hormones, testosterone, is extremely important in that it stimulates growth and sexual potency in both men and women. Higher testosterone levels found in women elicit a greater interest in sex, and increased orgasms. In aging men, as testosterone levels decline, there is a resulting commensurate loss of sex drive, premature ejaculation and the inability to maintain an erection. The hormone called leuteinizing hormone (LH) that is secreted by the pituitary gland, gives the signal for testosterone to be produced. Velvet antlers have high levels of LH and testosterone which stimulate the male testicle to convert cholesterol to testosterone.

Chinese doctors have used antler velvet for male incontinence, prostatic problems, and enlarged prostates for thousands of years. This may be attributed to other parts of the antler such as the anti-inflammatory prostaglandins and the anti-inflammatory portions of the cartilage. For women, besides helping with frigidity and infertility the antlers contain a high amount of calcium, useful in preventing osteoporosis. It may also help in the treatment of menstrual disorders.

Homeopathy

Agnus Castus (The Chaste Tree) is used when the sexual vitality is low in both sexes, but is more pronounced in men. For men it helps with erections, testicles and seminal fluid. With women, it relaxes the genitals, fear of sexual intimacy and scanty menstrual periods.

Sabal Serrulata (Saw Palmetto) is homeopathic to the irritability of the genito-urinary organs. It promotes nutrition and tissue building and is very valuable in treating prostatic enlargement. It builds up sexual power and aids in ejaculation. For women, sabal serrulata is valuable for undeveloped mammary glands, fear of sexual intimacy, and tender and enlarged ovaries

Cantharis relieves symptoms in men such as absence of normal erection, loss of vitality in sperm, weakness after ejaculation and temporary impotence or frigidity. For women, it rebalances menses.

Herbs

Herbs will not turn men into supermen, or make women love slaves, but herbs may be a good remedy choice when there are sexual dysfunctions. Normal sexual function requires healthy organs and balanced glands to produce sex hormones. Herbs, as superior body balancers, combine with our body and work through the glands. They are uniquely qualified to help achieve better gland response and overcome body deficiencies for a healthier sex life. Herbs may also work specifically, and are often quick to remedy sexual problems and enrich the sexual experience. The greatest benefit of using herbs for sexuality is that they work so individually with the human body. Herbal remedies are more successful when combined with other herbs. Here is how herbs work for men and women for sexual enhancement.

Herbs For Men:

• *Ashwagandha* has a long history in Ayurvedic history. It is very useful in cases of fatigue, calms the body down, lessens anxiety and increases sperm count.
• *Avena sativa* (wild and green oats) helps to increase stamina, strength and vitality along with increased

testosterone levels. It increases sexual desire and performance.

• *Cayenne pepper.* One of the most powerful natural circulatory stimulants, Cayenne red pepper gets the blood moving to everywhere it is needed, including the sex organs. "Cayenne puts lead in your pencil!" according to author Dick Quinn referring to the pepper's power to relieve sexual dysfunction. In his book, *Left for Dead*, Quinn chronicles the use of the hot herb for circulatory problems, ranging from heart disease and high blood pressure, to ulcers and impotence. The power of cayenne is measured in heat units. The culinary spice is only about 2,000 heat units whereas supplemental cayenne comes in 40-120,000 heat unit products. Dick Quinn suggests 2 capsules, 3 times a day to boost circulation.

• *Garlic* has been used as a natural remedy for centuries. It's been called the miracle herb as protection from virus, bacteria, parasites and fungus. Much research into the benefits of aged garlic extract (AGE) has been done AGE offers liver protection, prevents cancer, and acts as a free-radical fighter. Because of the compounds related to sex hormones, AGE may increase the sperm count in males. It is very helpful for stress reduction by lowering corticord, a hormone secreted by the body during stress. Garlic also helps to lower blood pressure, blood cholesterol levels, and acts as a tonic on the cardiovascular system.

• *Ginkgo biloba* is an important herb for strength, vitality, mental alertness and to enhance vitality levels. It improves the blood flow in small veins, and is extremely beneficial in the treatment of erectile dysfunction caused by lack of blood flow to the penis. Ginkgo also is a primary brain and mental energy stimulant, enhancing cerebral circulation.

• *Ginseng (Panax)* is perhaps the best known of the so-called aphrodisiac herbs. Research concludes that despite its reputation, it does not have a specific effect on the sexual organs. The plant has gained its reputation because of its ability to increase all-around well-being, stamina and endurance. As an adaptogenic (regulator) herb, ginseng helps the body deal with stress, increasing energy levels and decreasing fatigue. It does enhance male vitality, especially when in combination with herbs like Sarsaparilla and Damiana. Research has shown that ginseng contains plant testosterone and is the only known herb that can stimulate production of testosterone in the body. For men with an ailing prostate gland, ginseng appears to help healing and normalization of function. This herb also enhances nitric oxide synthesis, regulating the muscular tone of blood vessels to control blood flow to the penis, similar to the effect of popular drugs.

• *Kava Kava and Ginger* combination produces a mild euphoria and may be gently stimulating to the genital area. It also acts as a relaxant to reduce stress, which may improve the ability to reduce performance anxiety.

• *Maca* (Peruvian ginseng) has been used by the Incas for both nutritional and medicinal purposes. It is a nutritional powerhouse that is especially rich in iodine, amino acids, complex carbohydrates and essential minerals such as iron, zinc, phosphorus, calcium and magnesium. Maca also contains various vitamins such as B1, B2, B12, C and E. Maca enhances female fertility, increases energy, stamina in athletes, promotes mental clarity, treats male impotence, and helps with menstrual irregularities. It has been used to treat (female hormonal imbalances, including menopause) and chronic fatigue syndrome. Maca's reputed fertility enhancement may be due to its high content of iodine and zinc, amino acids and vitamin C.

• *Muira Puama* (potentwood) helps stimulate male libido and overcome erectile dysfunction. For women it's also used as a sexual enhancer for frigidity.

• *Pygeum africanum* is especially effective in inhibiting the production of prostaglandins in the prostate. It helps with inflammation, blood cholesterol and excess fluid in the prostate.

• *Sarsaparilla* is an excellent hormone balancing herb for both men and women. It contains the male hormone testosterone, progesterone and cortin which stimulate the action of estrogen in females.

• *Saw palmetto* is a natural steroid source herb with tissue building and gland stimulating properties to tonify and strengthen the male reproductive system. It is a primary herb for male impotence, low libido, and prostate health. The potency is increased when combined with another herb called Damiana, which also helps to increase sperm count. For women, it can be used as a mild aphrodisiac, to increase fertility and possibly enlarge underdeveloped breasts.

• *Similax officinalis* is a plant sterol that helps the body make testosterone. It comes from the root of the plant that has a flavoring called sarsaparilla. Similax helps lower cholesterol, and is very popular with body builders because it increases energy and endurance.

• *Tribulus terrestis* (puncture vine) is most commonly found in the Indian subcontinent and Africa. It has been used since ancient times in India as a treatment for sexual dysfunction. The most common cross-cultural use of the tribulus terrestis herb has been in the treatment of infertility in women, impotence in men and for increasing libido of both sexes. Tribulus appears to raise the testosterone production in men via the activation of leutinizing hormone (LH) secretion from the pituitary gland. The benefit of tribulus on the endocrine system and hormone production is believed to be largely due to its action in the liver. It acts as a liver tonic, improving the emulsification of fats to essential fatty acids, which along with cholesterol, is used by the liver to manufacture hormones.

• *Valerian root* is a strong, pain-relieving, safe sedative herb for anxiety, stress, PMS, menstrual cramping and emotional depression. It doesn't have the common side effects associated with narcotics used for similar purpose. It is an effected healer for the nervous system and can reduce anxiety associated with performance.

• *Yohimbe* is one of the most popular aphrodisiac herbs available. Dopamine (a neurotransmitter) levels decline in the brain as we age, causing sex drive and brain functions to drop. Yohimbe enhances the stimulation of neurotransmitters, which open the valve to the penis and causes more rapid and frequent erections. It has a reputation for producing electrifying sexual encounters. The aphrodisiac effects of Yohimbe are attributed to the enlargement of blood vessels in the sex organs and also to the increase reflexes in the lower region of the spinal cord. In practical terms, this increase in blood flow results in more rapid penile erections.

Herbs For Women:

• *Ashwagandha* is an Ayurvedic herb with ginseng-like activity that works well for women because it is a gentle energizer, less aggressive than panax ginseng, and well suited to a woman's needs. It helps increase female sexual energy without over-stimulating.

• *Avena sativa* (wild and green oats) is usually recommended for impotence and menstrual problems resulting from nervous exhaustion. It increases sexual desire and performance, with the possibilities of multiple orgasms.

• *Black cohosh* is used in female gland toning compounds for PMS, menstrual problems and menopausal symptoms. It helps increase fertility by regulating hormone production, especially after discontinuing the birth control pill.

• *Chaste Tree berry* helps normalize a woman's sex drive, stimulating production of progesterone by balancing abnormally high estrogen levels. It helps for depression, headaches, premenstrual acne, breast tenderness, cramps and bloating.

• *Damiana* has been found to contain several alkaloids that directly stimulate the nerves and sex organs, increase circulation and have muscle-relaxant properties. This herb helps treat frigidity in women and is a sexual energizer for both men and women. It is one of the most popular and safest of all herbs used to restore libido. Damiana works by increasing the messages sent throughout the nervous system, thereby increasing response to the sense of touch.

• *Dendrobium leaf* (Chinese Herb) helps nourish sensitive vaginal tissue by increasing body fluids. Combined with Licorice, it rebalances the hormonal levels.

• *Dong Quai* restores a woman to hormone harmony. Often called the "female ginseng" because it acts as an adaptogen (regulator) to maintain a woman's proper deep body balance. This herb may alleviate hot flashes and vaginal atrophy during menopause. This herb has been called the 'queen of all female herbs.'

• *False Unicorn* is a uterine tonic for infertility and frigidity that balances production of estrogen and progesterone.

• *Ginseng (Siberian)* help's restore a woman's body balance, both physically and biochemically. It helps preserve the health of female organs, especially in cases where natural estrogen is absent, such as following a hysterectomy, and prevents vaginal atrophy. It also modulates hormone release, improves fertility, boosts energy and relieves the irritability of pre-menopause and menopause.

• *Kava Kava combined with Ginger Root* increases blood flow to the extremities, including the genital area.

• *Licorice* contains traces of phytoestrogen sterols similar to those produced by the adrenal glands. It increases longevity and improves erotic arousal and stamina. Licorice has a normalizing effect on the body for fluid retention, breast tenderness, abdominal bloating, mood swings as well as depression.

• *Sarsaparilla* is an excellent hormone balancing herb for both men and women. It contains the male hormone testosterone, progesterone and cortin which stimulate the action of estrogen in females.

• *Tribulus terrestis* (puncture vine) is most commonly found in the Indian subcontinent and Africa. It has been used since ancient times in India as a treatment for sexual dysfunction. In women, follicle stimulating hormone (FSH) secretion and estrodial are increased. The most common cross-cultural use of the Tribulus terrestis herb has been in the treatment of infertility in women, impotence in men and for increasing libido of both sexes.

• *Wild yam* has hormone-like compounds that support the body's own hormone production. It is commonly used to offset symptoms experienced during menopause as well as reduce menstrual cramps, hormone-induced headaches, and PMS.

• *Yohimbe* is one of the most popular aphrodisiac herbs available. The aphrodisiac effects of Yohimbe are attributed to the enlargement of blood vessels in the sex organs and to the increases reflexes in the lower region of the spinal cord. In practical terms, this increase in blood flow results in more rapid penile erections. Yohimbe benefits female frigidity too, by stimulating blood flow to a woman's clitoris.

Vitamins

Select vitamins that aid in sexual dysfunction are listed below.

• *Bioflavonoids* support capillary blood flow, especially to the penis which aids in erectile capacity. They are important to healthy mucous membrane tissue and have estrogenic qualities.

• *Folic Acid* is a B vitamin that is an increasingly important supplement for pregnant women in preventing neural tube defects in fetuses. It is also helpful for ovarian function and sperm production.

• *Vitamin A*, an antioxidant, supports healthy adrenal function, which is important for sperm production and healthy mucous membrane tissue, like that of the vagina. A deficiency causes atrophy in sex organs, and may impair production of sex hormones.

• *Vitamin B3* may increase blood flow to the extremities. 100mg niacin, (not Niacinamide, which is not absorbed by the body) taken about 30 minutes before sex, may enhance sexual flush, mucous membrane tingling and the intensity of the orgasm.

• *Vitamin B5*, (pantothenic acid) supports adrenal function in forming steroid hormones, and provides pituitary support, thereby contributing to reducing male impotence and improving sexual stamina.

• *Vitamin B6* is involved in making neurotransmitters such as epinephrine which is thought to be involved in orgasm.

B6 also supports adrenal function, and may help male sex drive and impotence.

• *Vitamin B12* found in healthy sperm, may help impotence and support adrenal function.

• *Vitamin C* is important for sperm production and motility, and against impotence. For women, vitamin C is particularly key to the synthesis of hormones in the adrenal glands. The adrenals are designed to produce hormones that are converted to estrogen in body fat when ovarian hormone production slows down.

• *Vitamin E* is an antioxidant important for sperm production and has been used to treat male infertility. For women, this vitamin may be used both internally and topically, to relieve vaginal dryness. Massaging the inner sides of the vagina with vitamin E oil directly may help dry and damaged tissues. Succinate form of Vitamin E is better absorbed.

Flower remedies

Homeopathic preparations of flowering plants and trees have been known to alleviate many emotional and psychological problems. In cases of sexual inadequacies, feelings of failure, insecurity, irritation, and frustration may be lessened with the help of flower remedies. People with a feelings of inadequacies may be helped by flower essences of Elm, Larch, Larkspur, Saguaro Cactus and Wild Mountain Iris. Feelings of frustration can be helped by Chaparral, Daffodil, Impatiens, Lotus, Morning Glory, Potentilla, Wild Mountain Iris and Willow. These preparations are commonly administered by sublingual application (under the tongue) and can be found in most health food stores.

The ancient Chinese believe that an imbalance of physical sexual energy is normally caused by a lifelong loss of our sexual essence. Common physical causes of dwindling sexual desire include fatigue, depletion of yang (male) energy and ill health. Psychological factors include depression, anxiety, severe stress or a loss of a loved one. In Traditional Chinese Herbal Medicine, sexual impotence has various causes and needs a variety of herbal combinations to treat the problem.

One of these herbs is called, Horny Goat Weed or Goat Sex Herb. It has been used successfully for centuries by Chinese herbalists to improve sexual functions. It has androgen-like effects. Androgens are involved in sexual desire in both men and women. This herb is useful in stimulating sexual desire in women who are androgen deficient. Horny Goat Weed is a very strong and stimulating herb. It lowers blood pressure by dilating even the smallest capillaries as well as the major blood vessels of the circulatory system. An increase in the secretion of hormones is created almost immediately by this herb's strong alliance with the kidneys. A substantial increase in semen count and density has been recorded within the first few hours after ingestion.

Rhodiola Rosea, also known as Rosen Root and Golden Root, has been used for years in traditional Chinese folk medicine to increase mental alertness and acuity and to fight off fatigue. An additional benefit comes out of studies conducted on 35 patients suffering from premature ejaculation and/or weak erections. Upon a 3 month administration of Rhodiola extract, 26 patients reported significant improvement of sexual function and normalization in prostatic fluids.

Appendix

Stress Factors:

When the average person is under great stress for whatever reason, people compromise their eating habits. Instead of increasing the nutritious foods in their diet and adding necessary supplements, they eat fast foods, sugary snacks and drink alcohol. These contribute to depression, fatigue and aggravate their stressful condition. This also compromises their immune systems making them more susceptible to illness, including the common cold. Sometimes the mental state becomes so aggravated that they succumb to a diagnosis of mental illness. This can result in physicians prescribing an array of drugs. When our diets leave us in such straits, the last thing we think about is our sexuality. Our libido vanishes depriving us of one of natures most gratifying pleasures, and compounded with stress induced erectile failure, sets the stage for long lasting psychological impotence.

Upon the recognition of the first stages of stress, we should improve our diets immediately. Besides the good basic food structure that most people are aware of, we need to supplement with certain nutrients that will improve our mental outlook. The immune system must be supported prior to treatment for stress. Since the body has the ability to heal most of our ailments, we must give it the tools it needs to effect a cure. Adding extra minerals, enzymes and essential fatty acids to your diet, gives your body the basics. Additionally, you can add specific herbs and other nutrients that reduce stress.

Stress depletes the brain's neurotransmitters. When faced with a stressful situation, the brain uses large amounts of feel-good transmitters called endorphins. This upsets the ratio of many of the other transmitters creating a chemical imbalance in the body. The result is increased anxiety and a sense of urgency. When psychological or sexual problems cause stressful situations, amino acid supplementation is necessary in order to avoid aggravating the neurotransmitter imbalance and creating more stress. DL-phenylalanine and L-glutamine are key amino acids indicated in supporting neurotransmitter production which are keys to reducing stress.

Following is a list of supplements that may help in stress reduction.

Stress reduction supplementation suggestions:

• Amino acid supplement
• Lecithin granules
• Liquid crystalloid electrolyte minerals
• Digestive enzymes taken with meals
• Flaxseed (ground)
• St. John's Wort and Ashwagandha herbs
• Kava-Kava herbal tinctures
• Multi-vitamin supplement
• Ginseng tea
• Calcium-magnesium supplement (1:1 ratio)

• Additionally for men: Saw Palmetto extract or capsule
• Additionally for women: Don Quai extract

Dosages vary depending on individuals, therefore we recommend consulting a health practitioner schooled in natural methods of preventive medicine.

Chapter 5
Resource Directory.

YOHIMBE POWER. *Yohimbe Power Max™ 2000* for men, is one of the most potent sources of Yohimbe Bark Extract available. Each dose features 2,000 mg. of pure Yohimbe Bark Extract, the ultimate formula for power and performance. *Avena Sativa* (Wild Oats) is a high potency energizing herbal tonic for men and women with research showing its stimulating effects in restoring and heightening sexual performance, strength and stamina. *Ginseng Power Max® 4X* for men and women features four standardized Ginseng herbal extracts: Chinese, Korean, Siberian and American synergistically blended into one power-packed formula that provides daily optimum energy support. ACTION LABS, 280 Adams Blvd. Farmingdale, NY 11735   (800) 932-2953   fax (516) 694-6493

NATURAL ESTROVEN—To maintain a woman's balance. Based on natural estrogens from soy and other plants, daily dietary supplementation with *ESTROVEN* helps provide a natural hormonal balance and may ease fluctuating estrogen levels in women, which can begin in their mid 30's. A deficiency of estrogen can result in vaginal dryness and thinning of the vaginal walls - both of which can interfere with the pleasure of sexual intercourse. *ESTROVEN* provides 50 mg. of soy and plant estrogens in each daily caplet, and also includes balancing vitamins and minerals including B6, B12 and folic acid, calcium for bones and natural Vitamin E. *ESTROVEN*, normally taken in the evening or prior to bedtime also includes kava kava, the traditional calming herb. AMERIFIT, INC., 166 Highland Park Drive, Bloomfield, CT 06002 (800) 990-3476 http://www.estroven.com

ADD EXCITEMENT TO INTIMATE MOMENTS. All body functions need proper nutrient support for optimal sexual performance. *Love Male*, featuring Yohimbe bark, offers a powerful and potent herbal blend designed to improve peak sexual performance, enhance stamina and increase virility and libido. *Love Female* removes the low energy component for the loss of sexual desire and helps balance hormone levels needed to promote a healthy libido, and support heightened levels of pleasure. *Women's Dryness,* contains Dendrobium Leaf to help nourish sensitive vaginal tissue by increasing body fluids. Licorice Root helps balance hormonal levels. CRYSTAL STAR HERBAL NUTRITION, 4069 Wedgeway Court, Earth City, MO 63045   (800) 736-6015

REJUVENATE YOUR CIRCULATION. Cayenne Trading Company offers circulation-boosting herb formulas, *Cayenne King, Golden Garlic, Hawthorn Heart Quinn's Blend All-in-One, Red Bird and American Energy.* Also available is certified organic Canadian Flaxseed provided by fast service. A free catalog and newsletter is available by calling us. CAYENNE TRADING CO., 114 Minnesota Ave., Sebeka, MN 56477   (800) 641-6802

VIRILITY ENHANCING FORMULA. Deepak's *LIBIDOPLEX* contains the broadest spectrum of virility enhancing extracts and essential vitamins available, including 28 ingredients specially formulated to benefit the reproductive system of both men and women. In addition to their libido-enhancing effects, several ingredients have been shown to reduce the risk of prostate cancer in men, and are a safe alternative to drug therapies available today. For catalogue information contact: DEEPAK'S NATURAL REMEDIES, LLC, (800) 200-0456 or visit our Internet site: http://www.deepak.com

FRESH FROM THE FARM. FLAX FOR YOUR IMMUNE SYSTEM. A whole food, *Dakota Flax Gold* is all natural edible fresh flax seed, is high in lignins which can be used over cereal, on salads, in soups or in juice. Ready to grind, just like your best coffee, it is low in cadmium and is better tasting than packaged flax products. Seeds must be ground for full nutritional value. Dakota Flax Gold is available with grinder. Flax, also available in capsule form as *Flaxeon Jet,* is a convenient way of getting beneficial essential fatty acids. HEINTZMAN FARMS, RR2 Box 265, Onaka SD 57466   (800) 333-5813   (send S.A.S.E. for sample) http://www.heintzmanfarms.com

ALL NATURAL ALTERNATIVE FOR IMPOTENCY. *RexHard* is a blend of essential nutrients, vitamins, minerals and amino acids combined with potent herbal extracts. *RexHard* improves desire, performance and firmness for increased sexual pleasure. It increases energy and circulation. Erotic Tea is an exotic blend for men and women who wish to enjoy an active sexual lifestyle. *CholestoPlex* and *CardioPlex* offer nutritional support for healthy cholesterol levels and a healthy strong heart which are important factors for a satisfying sex life. MAMAR LABS, INC., 4646 Domestic Ave. #101, Naples FL 34104   (800) 862-3931 Email: mamar33@aol.com   http://www.mamar-labs.com

VELVET ANTLER CAPSULES. Historically, v*elvet antler* has been used for more than 2,000 years. Since velvet antler is said to build up the body's natural resources, many consider it one of the most versatile all around health food supplements, and is becoming known as nature's perfect food. Known in Asia through ancient medicine as an aphrodisiac, velvet antler is known for its gonadotropic activity and sexual enhancement. The elk are raised on farms in North America and the velvet antler harvested annually without causing harm to the animal. It is processed and then encapsulated at a FDA inspected laboratory. MEADOW CREEK ELK FARMS, 7860 Woodland Lane, West Bend, WI 53090 (800)547-8450#01   http://www.hnet.net/~elkacres

CRYSTALLOID ELECTROLYTE MINERALS. *Trace-Lyte™* liquid is a crystalloid (smallest form) electrolyte formula that helps keep cells strong, balance pH, facilitate removal of toxins and provide the body's life force. If extra magnesium is required, *Cal-Lyte™* offers a 1:1 ratio of calcium/magnesium with boron to assist absorption. Also available is *Total-Lyte™* which increases mental efficiency, improves concentration, nourishes the brain and combats fatigue. NATURE'S PATH, INC., PO Box 7862, Venice, FL 34287-7862   (800)-326-5772.

HEIGHTEN SEXUAL PROWESS. Among its many properties, bee pollen has the ability to help maintain the integrity of the cell, and foster immune support. Plus, in years past, bee pollen has shown great power in restoring body functioning including the rebuilding of the reproductive system. *Pollen-Lyte* provides bee pollen together with crystalloid electrolytes for maximum utilization in the body. *Bio-Lyte* contains bioflavonoids that prevent arteries from hardening, and enhance blood vessels, capillary and vein strength. They also help lower cholesterol and stimulate bile production. NATURE'S PATH, INC., P.O. Box 7862, Venice FL 34287-7862   (800) 326-5772

SEX & NATURAL HORMONE THERAPY.
Symbiotropin™ (a Growth Hormone Releaser) was shown clinically to increase sexual potency/frequency by 32% and duration of penile erection by 44% within 90 days. *Testron SX*™ contains a variety of natural compounds to help support testosterone production. Safe and effective, it may be used by men and women for increased virility. For more information contact: NUTRACEUTICS CORP., 3317 NW Tenth Terrace, Suite 404, Fort Lauderdale, FL 33309
(800) 391-0114 (east coast)   (800) 852-8582 (west coast)

SPANISH FLY HOMEOPATHIC REMEDY. *Spanish Fly* helps to normalize sexual sensitivities for both the male and female. These include loss of desire and dysfunction and impotence due to stress. *Spanish Fly* homeopathic remedy includes Agnus castus, Cantharis, Staphysagria, Sabal 15x, Echinacea, Sabal, Hydrastis, Urtica urens, Thuja, Gaultheria, and Ginseng 3x. Use in combination with *#1 DETOXIFIER* complex is necessary. NEWTON LABORATORIES, 2360 Rockaway Industrial Blvd., Conyers, GA 30012
(800)-448-7256   http/:www.newtonlabs.net

FORMULAS FOR DESIRE AND STAMINA. Hormonal changes, lifestyle stress and fatigue can reduce a woman's sexual impulses. *Women's Natural Desire* contains a unique blend of herbs, including Yohimbe, Ginseng, Damiana, Dong Quai and Wild Yam Root for a women's most intimate moments. This all-natural women's supplement may help add excitement to your sex life and increase your sexual desire. Women's Natural Products is a trusted name in women's supplements. For men, the all-natural *Male Drive*™ men's supplement contains Yohimbe and Ginseng to help improve stamina, pleasure and sexual performance. NUTRITION NOW®, INC., P.O. Box 6249, Vancouver, WA 98668-6249
(800) 929-0418

MACA. Called the "Peruvian Ginseng" from the Andes, is a tuber that is traditionally used for virility, impotency and fertility. Traditionally *Maca* has also been used for increased energy, stamina and athletic endurance. It is also available in a formula called *INVIGOR-X*™ which includes maca, American and Siberian ginseng bound with *CRYSTALLOID ELECTROLYTES. BODY-X*™ is a phyto-nutrient rich body lotion designed to feed and nurture the skin. Nutrient oils and herbal extracts are combined to provide smoother skin. NUTRAMEDIX, INC., 212 U.S. Hwy #1, Suite 17, Tequesta, FL 33469   (800) 742-2529   http://www.nutramedix.com

HERBAL HORMONE ACTIVATOR, T2. Tribulus terrestris appears to act as a hormone activator. Increased fertility and libido are some results of this action. For more information on T2 and other hormone potentiators call NUTRITIONAL TECH., INC., The science behind nutrition is here. San Diego, CA 92111
(888) 300-0707 Email:NTIHO@aol.com   http://www.nticorp.com

ENZYMES FOR IMMUNE SUPPORT. The lack of enzymes in our cooked-food diets hamper proper digestion. This limits the nutrient absorption needed by our bodies to support our immune system. *TYME ZYME*™, an all natural SCIENTIFICALLY PROVEN formula contains all the necessary enzymes for digestion throughout the intestinal tract. It contains protease, amylase, lipase, cellulase and lactase. When taken with meals, it increases nutrient absorption and assures the body of receiving the benefits of vital nutrients, especially zinc, selenium and essential fatty acids. This strengthens the immune system, aids in digestion and increases energy. PROZYME PRODUCTS, LTD., (800) 522-5537 call Debra Casey for information.

SEXUAL ENHANCEMENT WITH AROMA. The special *Aromance Blend* and seven custom House Blends made from pure therapeutic grade essential oils, are available for use in inhalation, bath and massage. Products include guide sheets for usage. *The Oil Lady Aromatherapy Medicine Tin* of essential oils is also available with a guide booklet. OIL LADY AROMATHERAPY®, 764 12TH Avenue South, Naples, FL 34102   (941) 263-3451
Fax (941) 263-0898

BRAIN FOOD FOR YOUR SEX LIFE. As necessary ingredients for proper cellular neurotransmitter function in the brain and circulation throughout the body, Omega-3 essential fatty acids must be balanced with Omega-6 essential fatty acids. Flax provides a good balance of these nutrients. *Fortified Flax* contains Organic Flax seed, Zinc, Vitamin B-6, C, E and is "yeast free". For a healthy snack, they also offer flax in a tasty *Omega Bar*, a convenient way to get your energy. *Fortified Flax* and *Power Pack Energy Drink Mix* can be mixed in juice or water or it can be sprinkled on salads, cereal or sandwiches. OMEGA-LIFE, INC., P.O. Box 208, Brookfield, WI 53008-0208   (800) EAT-FLAX (328-3529)

STRENGTHEN YOUR STAMINA. *Pines Wheat Grass* and *Barley Grass* tablets are a convenient and natural way to get nutrients your body needs. In addition to naturally occurring vitamins, minerals, amino acids, protein, enzymes and chlorophyll, Pines International's cereal grasses contain fiber which may aid in promoting regularity. *Mighty Greens*, a synergistic blend of superfoods, designed to provide high-quality nutrition and contains herbs which may assist in relief of minor fatigue. PINES INTERNA-TIONAL, INC., P.O. Box 1107, Lawrence, KS 66044
(800) 697-4637   http://www.wheatgrass.com

SPROUTED SOY SUPPLEMENT AND PROGESTERONE CREAM. *REGENEZYME* powder (or caplets) is an all natural 100% organic, sprouted whole food concentrate. Sprouted soy does not contain the same allotype of provocative allergens common to soybean products. It is an excellent source of isoflavones and is beneficial to prostate health, menopausal symptoms and protein deficient diets. *ENDOCREME* serum or cream is a transdermal (percutaneous) delivery of natural progesterone and hormone precursors. These beneficial substances are more bioavailable to the body than in an orally used form.—especially due to *Endocreme's* proprietary delivery system ("Invisible Patch"). The products contain whole plant extracts, to provide a more synergistic and balancing effect.. SEDNA SPECIALTY HEALTH PRODUCTS, P.O. Box 1453, Andrews, NC 28901 (800) 223-0858

TRANSFORMATION ENZYME FORMULAS.
Proper nutrition and absorption play an important factor in improving sexual dysfunction. *DigestZyme* provides high potency multiple enzymes to help digest food nutrients. *PureZyme* purifies the blood and lymphatic systems. Because the lymphatic system carries away toxins from all body cells and the blood delivers oxygen and nutrients to all cells and organs, their proper function is crucial to the health of the entire body. *Plantadophilus* balances the pH in the colon and throughout the intestines. It also acts as a natural antibiotic further strengthening the immune system. TRANSFORMATION, 2900 Wilcrest, Suite 220, Houston, TX 77042   (800) 777-1474

CRANIOSACRAL THERAPY. *CranioSacral Therapy* is a gentle method of evaluating and enhancing the craniosacral system, the environment in which the brain and spinal cord function. Developed by John E. Upledger, D.O., O.M.M., this light touch manual therapy encourages the body's natural healing mechanisms to improve the capability of the central nervous system. It also encourages the negative effects of stress to dissipate, strengthens resistance to disease and enhances health. Call for information or to order an international directory of practitioners: THE UPLEDGER INSTITUTE HEALTHPLEX CLINICAL SERVICES, 11211 Prosperity Farms Rd., D-223, Palm Beach Gardens, FL 33410-3487 (561) 622-4706

GINKGO AND GARLIC. *Ginkgo Biloba Plus®* is a combination of *Kyolic®* aged garlic extract, ginkgo biloba extract and Siberian ginseng extract. This unique formula has proven to enhance brain power, resulting in more positive thinking, energized mental clarity and promotes a sense of well-being. Ginkgo is known to increase circulation throughout the body, especially to the sex organs. *Kyolic®* aged garlic extract enhances the immune system better than raw garlic. For free samples and literature please call or write to: WAKUNAGA OF AMERICA, 23501 Madero, Mission Viejo, CA 92692   (800) 825-7888

BOOST PERFORMANCE. Through herbs, nature has created potentially exciting substances for supporting human performance, brain function and sexual energy. *VIPP™ for Men* uses only the highest quality herbal extracts (Avena sativa, Yohimbe, Saw Palmetto and Siberian Ginseng) along with Niacin, DHEA and Pregnenolone. *VIPP™ for Women* contains specific herbs (Tribulus, Dong Quai, Avena sativa and Wild Yam) and Niacin and Vitamin B6 that support women's bodies. Combined with today's science of formulation these synergistic blends surpass all others. WASHBROOKS, 190 Beach St., Laguna Beach, CA 92651 (888) 674-4543

SUPER BLUE GREEN® ALGAE. *Mazama Mix*, a green drink includes a wide variety of sprouted organically grown grains and grasses. providing an unequaled combination of whole foods, from all-natural sources. It provides a balanced source fiber that allows your body to utilize food for energy. It supplies complete protein and all of the amino acids used by the body to create muscles, antibodies and lean connective tissues. *Mazama Mix* also includes powerful nutritional plant-based enzymes, which enhance digestive function. Coupled with *Alpha & Omega Sun* algae, your body will react with higher stamina and increased energy levels. This food will help strengthen your immune system, reduce stress, anxiety and depression. For free audio tape & information: Bill & Terri Edwards, Independent Distributors, P.O. Box 626, Pine Lake, GA 30072 (800) 927-2527 ext. 06144   Email: PWPT32A@prodigy.com

HORNY GOAT WEED FORMULA. All natural herbal alternative to prescription drugs. *Horny Goat Weed Formula™* is a unique and extremely potent blend of herbs, specially coated to stop stomach acid from destroying their nutrients. This formula includes Mucuna Pruriens Extract (20% L-Dopa), Muira Puama Extract, Tribulus Terrestris Extract and Horny Goat Weed. These potent individual herbs have been used by healers to enhance performance, promote endurance, restore desire and powerful urges, and increase erectile ability. For women that have had hysterectomies, the benefits are similar. Also available, *TRIPLE STRENGTH GROWTH HORMONE™*, an all natural Ayurvedic herbal formula. This special synergistic blend of herbal extracts combined with a unique delivery system, produces a very potent and extremely effective growth hormone enhancer. FOUNTAIN OF YOUTH, Inc., 6811 Tylersville Rd., Ste 167, W. Chester OH 45069 (800) 939-4296

AROUSAL CREAM. Optimal erections, naturally with *Arousal™*, a safer and far less expensive alternative to prescription drugs. Contains natural L-Arginine (an essential amino acid) in a break through trans-dermal delivery cream that some say restores and enhances normal erectile function. Also available is *Sensation for Women™* for what could be full sexual response and heightened pleasure, naturally. Contains the natural amino acid L-Arginine, proven to heighten the sexual response, improving orgasms and the ease in which they are achieved. Both products come in a translucent gel, scent-free and undetectable. NATURAL PLEASURES, P.O. Box 6430, Whittier, CA 90609 (888) 447-8600 www.naturalpleasure.com

FLOWER ESSENCES, Deva Flower Remedy®, *Inadequacy/Failure* is designed to help those who lack confidence in their abilities and for those who fear failure. It could help to connect one to his or her own power, to take a stand, be forward and straight, more self confident and be courageous and emotionally strong. *Frustration/Irritation* treats those who are impatient, irritable, restless, blocked, annoyed, on edge or have insomnia. Formulated to help balance the mental body from disturbing and conflicting thoughts helping one to stay centered. NATURAL LABS CORP., PO Box 20037, Sedona, AZ 86341 (800) 233-0810 Email: Natbio@sedona.net

HOMEOPATHIC GROWTH HORMONE. *Hormonegentic™* hand succussed homeopathic Growth Hormone (GH) 2C/30C. After age 25-30, levels of GH decline and that is when sexual function begins to decrease and general aging signs appear. One study on GH by Dr.'s Chein and Terry report that sexual potency and frequency increased 75% and duration of penile erection increased 62%. Clinical studies show men and women benefit not only sexually but with increased stamina, energy, strength, reduced wrinkles and fat, increase of lean tissue and toned muscle mass, improved eyesight, etc. *Hormonegentic™* is the highest quality homeopathic GH available. Homeopathics are safe, gentle and free of side effects. DREAMOUS CORP USA, 12016 Wilshire Blvd, #8, Los Angeles, CA 90025 (800) 251-7543   www.dreamous.com

AMORÉ-LYTE. Finally, a natural health product that delivers what it promises. This supplement will do more for the male libido than any other. Amoré-Lyte actually can restore the libido to its fullest capacity. And, there are NO side effects. This is truly a totally natural formula that works. Another fantastic feature of this unique product is the addition of crystalloid electrolytes, which both act as a synergistic factor for the libido and, through a process known as biovection, the electrolytes act as a super carrier of the nutrients to the body's cells. NATURE'S PATH INC., PO Box 7862, Venice, FL 34287-7862   (800)-326-5772.

MAIL ORDER CATALOG. *Omega Nutrition's mail order catalogue* carries many of the items recommended in "Natural Solutions for Sexual Enhancement," fresh from the farm and organic. Flax seeds, Essential Fatty Acid supplements including flax oil, Saw Palmetto Plus (with Pygeum,) Zinc, Vitamin E, hGH secretagogues, Royal Jelly, Gingko, Ginseng, Chromium, Natural Progesterone creams, Electrolytes, Enzymes and more. One stop shopping with reasonable prices.To receive a free catalog call (800) 661-FLAX (661-3529).

SPROUTED SOY CAPSULES. *Soy Guard*™ a concentrated 'live' soy supplement, retains the sprouts precious phytochemicals, enzymes, vitamins and minerals. Soy contains isoflavones, also know as phytoestrogens because they are similar in structure to natural estrogen although only $1/1000^{th}$ the strength. Excessive estrogen levels can be harmful, but these weak estrogens provide a positive effect on the body's natural estrogen and exhibit powerful anti-cancer effects in hormone related malignancies including breast cancer. Strong evidence indicates that Isoflavones in soy can block the negative effects of androgens on the prostate in men, thereby preventing enlargement and prostate cancer. BIOTEC FOODS, 5152 Bolsa Ave., Suite 101, Huntington Beach, CA 92649 (800) 788-1084

STRESS REDUCTION NEUROTRANSMITTER SUPPORT. *Restores*™ for adults and children contain the specific nutrients the brain must have to *replenish* low levels of vital neurotransmitters, a key element in reducing stress and improving brain function.. Made up of a special synergistic natural formulation of amino acids, vitamins and minerals, *Restores* also promotes increased seratonin, dopamine and endorphin levels. NUTRI-PET RESEARCH/Quest IV Health, 8 West Main St., Farmingdale, NJ 07727 (800) 360-3300

ALL NATURAL hGH PRECURSOR *Unitropin*™ contains natural substances that cause the pituitary gland to secrete human growth hormone (hGH). *Unitropin*™ is based on research revealed by Dr. Ronald Klatz, M.D., who states that amino acids and some B vitamins cause the pituitary to release hGH. *Unitropin*™ combines the scientifically proven benefits of hGH research: B vitamins, including Niacin, B6 and B12, amino acids including choline, L-Arginine, L-Ornithine, L-Tyrosine, DL-Methionine, Alpha Ketoglutarate and Melatonin with co-enzyme Q-10 and crystalloid electrolytes. *Unitropin*™ also contains a powerful, unique life-enhancing blend of herbs and extracts to improve sexual stamina and pleasure for both men and women. These include tribulus terrestris (to increase libido, recovery time from sexual activity, strength of erections and increase self-confidence in both men and women). It also contains Muira puama (a powerful aphrodisiac, nerve stimulant and overall mood enhancer), Korean Ginseng and Ashwaganda (that reduce stress and bring the body into a state of equilibrium.) These ingredients create a powerful "global" formula that effects both body and mind creating a synergistic sense of well being. UNIVERSAL NETWORK, INC., 5647 Beneva Road, Sarasota, FL 34332 (800) 446-0302   www. unitropin.com

INCREASE STAMINA AND PHYSICAL PERFORMANCE. 100% certified organic and Kosher wheat grass juice powder. *Sweet Wheat*® is pure green energy direct from nature. High in zinc and vitamin A, vital to a healthy prostate gland for men and necessary to promote a healthy hormonal balance in women. It contains live enzymes for better digestion. *Sweet Wheat* also helps skin and eyesight as well as fortifying the immune system. This formula enhanced with crystalloid electrolytes is available as *Electra Green.* SWEET WHEAT, P.O. Box 187, Clearwater, FL 33757-0187 (888) 227-9338   www.SweetWheat.com

Epilog.

Sex is a form of communication and communion. In order to create this union, sex has to unfold with no time line or expectations. One needs to appreciate all aspects of one's sexuality from the exquisite ability to attract others, to being able to partake in any degree of sexual contact and expression without any "strings attached".

Love pulls us with a magnetic force toward unity and wholeness. When a relationship blossoms into love, the sexual act of giving and receiving erotic pleasure, emotional nourishment and spiritual oneness with our loved one becomes a fundamental human expression. Sexual fulfillment may provide ultimate joy in sharing intimacy, orgasm and love. Loving sex may bring with it a supreme source of mutual healing and awakening of the spirit. Sexual closeness generates a potent healing energy, restorative and nurturing for each partner.

Do you want to have a baby? Below is a suggested formula for men and women who are having a difficult time of conceiving.

"FERTILITY FORMULA"

Crystalloid Electrolytes: 6 teaspoons per day
Zinc: 15 mg. one per day
Nutritional Yeast: 3 tablets in morning and 3 in afternoon.
Vitamin E: 400IU supplement one per day
Wheat Germ Oil: 1/2 tablespoon per day
CranioSacral Therapy session (optional)

♥ Good Luck and God Bless!

Bibliography

-Anderson, Nina and Peiper, Howard, *Over 50 Looking 30, The Secrets of Staying Young*, Safe Goods, E. Canaan, CT, 1996

-Anderson, Nina and Peiper, Dr. Howard, *Crystalloid Electrolytes*, Safe Goods, E. Canaan, CT, 1998

-Baum, Neil, M.D., *Overcoming Impotence*, Delicious Magazine, June, 1998

-Bricklin, Mark, *The Practical Encyclopedia of Natural Healing*, Rodale Press, Inc. Emmaus, PA, 1976

-Brody, Jane E., *Do You Need The Hormone of Desire?* New York Times, Feb. 24, 1998

-Dunas, Felice PhD, *Passion Play*, Riverhead Books, NewYork, NY, 1997

-Fennessy, P.F., *Velvet antler: the product and pharmacology*, Proc. Deer Course for Veterinarians (Deer Branch of the NZ Vet. Association,) 1991

-Gittleman, Ann Louise, *Super Nutrition For Men*, M. Evans and Co. Inc., New York, NY, 1996

-Green, James, *The Male Herbal*, Crossing Press, Freedom, CA, 1991

-Jamieson, James, Dorman, Dr. L.E. and Marriott, Valerie, *Growth Hormone, The Methusalah Factor*, Safe Goods, E. Canaan, CT, 1997

-Kaptchuk, T. and Croucher, M., *The Healing Arts: Exploring the Medical Ways of the World*, Summit Books, New York, NY, 1987

-Kennedy, Lou, *A Pill to Regain Potency. Viagra*, Healthy Living, Sarasota FL, July 1998

-Kulvinskas, Viktoras, *The Lover's Diet*, Ihopea, Inc., Hot Springs, AR, 1998

-Lark, Susan M., M.D., *Safe Passage*, Delicious Magazine, July, 1998

-Lee, John, M.D., *Natural Progesterone: The multiple roles of A Remarkable Hormone*, BLI Publishing, Sebastopol, CA 1993

-Martlew, Gillian, *Electrolytes, The Spark of Life*, Nature's Publishing, North Port, FL, 1995

-Page, Dr. Linda, *Healthy Healing Guide to Sexuality*, Healthy Healing Publications, Carmel Valley, CA, 1998

-Page, Linda, Dr. *Super Drugs -"Youth in a Bottle" or a Life Sentence?*, Healthy Healing Updates & Natural Healing Solutions, June 1998

-Pearson, Durk and Shaw, Sandy, *Life Extension*, Warner Books, New York, NY, 1981

-Pizzorno, Joseph and Murray, Michael T., *Encyclopedia of Natural Medicine*, Prima Publishing, Rocklin, CA, 1998

-Thomas, John, *Young Again!* Plexus, Press, Kelso, WA, 1994

-Wade, Carlson, *Bee Pollen and Your Health*, Keats Publishing, New Canaan, CT 1978

-Watson, Cynthia, *Love Potions*, Putnam Publishing, Los Angeles, CA, 1993

-Weiner, Michael and Mill, Janet, *Herbs that Heal*, Quantum, Books Valley, CA, 1988

-Williams, L., *CLA*, Woodstock Publishing, Pleasant Grove, UT, 1997

INDEX

Authors:

Dr. Howard Peiper

Howard is a nationally recognized expert in the holistic counseling field. His healing, health care and natural health professional credentials extend over a thirty year period and include those of naturopath, author, lecturer, magazine consultant, radio personality and host of a television show, Partners in Healing Howard is the co-author of 10 books on alternative health and preventive care. He holds a degree in Optometry and now practices in the field of Naturopathy. For twenty years he has committed himself to the holistic field.

Nina Anderson

Nina is a nationally acclaimed researcher, author and lecturer. She is a former corporate jet pilot and is a consultant to the building industry where she specializes in non-toxic applications for housing. She has been an active researcher in the holistic health field for over twenty years and has co-authored 12 books primarily focusing on sickness prevention for both people and pets. Nina has a Bachelor's Degree from Monmouth College and is currently president of Safe Goods and the non-profit Scientific Alliance for Education.

OTHER BOOKS AVAILABLE FROM SAFE GOODS

★*A.D.D. The Natural Approach* $ 4.95
Alternatives to drug therapy for children and adults with attention deficit disorder.

★*Crystalloid Electrolytes* $ 4.95
Our body's energy source for the new millennium

★*The Brain Train* $ 4.95
How to keep our brain healthy and wise (for children).

★*Feeling Younger with Homeopathic HGH* $ 4.95
For everyone who wants to stay young at any age

★*All Natural Anti-Aging Skin Care* $ 4.95
The newest information on keeping your skin young.

★*The All Natural Anti-Aging Diet* $ 4.95
Eat lots, Stay slim and avoid old age diseases

★*Plain English Guide to your PC* $ 8.95
The computer book that tells it better and tells it in English.

★*A Guide To A Naturally Healthy Bird* $ 8.95
Nutritional information for parrots and other caged birds.

★*OVER 50 LOOKING 30! The Secrets of Staying Young.* $ 9.95
How to become wrinkle resistant and fight the signs of aging.

★*The A.D.D. and A.D.H.D. DIET!* $ 9.95
look at contributing factors and natural treatments for ADD/ADHD.

★*The Backseat Flyer* $ 9.95
Plane sense about flying as a passenger

★*Super Nutrition for Animals (Birds Too!)* $12.95
Healthy advice for Dogs, Cats, Ferrets, Horses and Birds.

★*Growth Hormone, The Methuselah Factor* $12.95
Reverse human aging naturally

★*Put Hemorrhoids & Constipation Behind You* $14.95
A natural healing guide for easy, quick, lasting relief

★*The Humorous Herbalist* $14.95
Practical guide to leaves, flowers, roots, bark and other neat stuff

Order Line (800)-903-3837
Safe Goods Publishing
PO Box 36, East Canaan, CT 06024
http://www.animaltails.com